It is important to note that absence of evidence of effectiveness does not imply absence of effectiveness.

Tables of systematic up-to-date reviews

Where systematic reviews of treatments were available they were summarized and included in table format. Treatments had to be beneficial or likely to be beneficial and up-to-date (i.e. recent or not contradicting evidence subsequently published) in order to be included.

Safety issues

The precautionary principle has been applied, i.e. a treatment is not considered risk-free unless evidence suggests otherwise; this is particularly pertinent to pregnancy and lactation which are cited as contraindications for all medicines. Only direct risks are listed i.e. any indirect risks such as inadequately trained practitioners, or delay of effective treatment are not included.

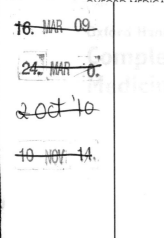

OXFORD MEDICAL PUBLICATIONS

Oxford Handbook of
Complementary
Medicine

OF01032

Books should be returned to the SDH Library on or before
the date stamped above unless a renewal has been arranged

Salisbury District Hospital Library

Telephone: Salisbury (01722) 336262 extn. 4432 / 33

Out of hours answer machine in operation

Oxford Handbook of
Complementary Medicine

Edzard Ernst MD PhD FRCP FRCPEd

Professor of Complementary Medicine
Peninsula Medical School
Universities of Exeter and Plymouth
Exeter, UK

Max H Pittler MD PhD

Senior Research Fellow in Complementary Medicine
Peninsula Medical School
Universities of Exeter and Plymouth
Exeter, UK

Barbara Wider MA

Research Fellow in Complementary Medicine
Peninsula Medical School
Universities of Exeter and Plymouth
Exeter, UK

Kate Boddy MA

Information Officer in Complementary Medicine
Peninsula Medical School
Universities of Exeter and Plymouth
Exeter, UK

OXFORD
UNIVERSITY PRESS

OXFORD
UNIVERSITY PRESS

Great Clarendon Street, Oxford OX2 6DP

Oxford University Press is a department of the University of Oxford.
It furthers the University's objective of excellence in research, scholarship,
and education by publishing worldwide in

Oxford New York

Auckland Cape Town Dar es Salaam Hong Kong Karachi
Kuala Lumpur Madrid Melbourne Mexico City Nairobi
New Delhi Shanghai Taipei Toronto

With offices in

Argentina Austria Brazil Chile Czech Republic France Greece
Guatemala Hungary Italy Japan Poland Portugal Singapore
South Korea Switzerland Thailand Turkey Ukraine Vietnam

Oxford is a registered trade mark of Oxford University Press
in the UK and in certain other countries

Published in the United States
by Oxford University Press Inc., New York

British Library Cataloguing in Publication Data

Data available

Library of Congress Cataloging in Publication Data

Data available

Typeset by Newgen Imaging Systems (P) Ltd., Chennai, India
Printed in Italy
on acid-free paper by
LegoPrint

ISBN 978–0–19–920677–3 (flexicover: alk.paper)

10 9 8 7 6 5 4 3 2 1

Foreword

About twenty years ago I was having a drink in a bar in Dublin with Petr Skrabanek, an iconoclast friend who made many important critical observations about medical practice. Two of the icons that were favourite targets for Petr were cancer screening programmes within orthodox medicine, and complementary medicine. Not long previously, an article of Petr's entitled 'Acupuncture and the age of unreason' had been published in *The Lancet* (Skrabanek 1984). I asked him how he had felt able to dismiss acupuncture so confidently without reviewing systematically the empirical evidence about its possible effects. Would it not be more appropriate to keep a more open mind about the worth of acupuncture until he had done that? I referred specifically to a randomised trial, reported by an internationally respected French research group, which had shown that gastroscopy in 90 patients had been much easier and better tolerated after real acupuncture than after placebo acupuncture (Cahn et al. 1978). "Iain", he said, "your mind is so open that your brains are falling out."

Petr Skrabanek's response to the positive results of a controlled experiment designed to evaluate the effects of one form of complementary medicine illustrates an all-too-common stance adopted by critics of complementary medicine: "Never mind if the empirical evidence suggests it works, the theory underpinning the practice is simply unbelievable". Yet orthodox medicine has made some catastrophic mistakes by basing practice solely on theory, as well as some major advances based on empirical observations unexplained by theory (see www.jameslindlibrary.org). So why don't the critics of complementary medicine acknowledge that reliable empirical evidence of beneficial effects should be the basis for distinguishing useful treatments from the other sort? Surely intellectual honesty demands a single standard of evidence across the board (Chalmers 1998).

Even if that logic is accepted, it leaves open the issue of what constitutes "reliable empirical evidence". People are bound to vary in what they regard as reliable evidence, and a leap of faith will always be required to make causal inferences about treatment effects. I tried to illustrate this some years ago in an article entitled 'What do I want from health research and researchers when I am a patient?' (Chalmers 1995). I noted that my wife began to believe that chiropractic could help relieve her chronic shoulder and back pain after about five treatments from a chiropractor, to whom she had been referred by her general practitioner. Although I was delighted that her longstanding symptoms had subsided, I did not begin to share her belief that chiropractic might have been responsible until a couple of years later when I read the report of a systematic review of the relevant controlled trials (Koes 1991).

For me and, I suspect, many others, 'reliable evidence' about the effects of health care will usually mean evidence derived from systematic reviews of carefully controlled evaluative research. Edzard Ernst and his colleagues at the Peninsula Medical School have done a great service by endeavouring to meet the need for such evidence in the 'Oxford Handbook of Complementary Medicine'.

Iain Chalmers
Editor, *James Lind Library*

References

Cahn AM, Carayon P, Hill C, Flamant R. Acupuncture in gastroscopy. Lancet. 1978;**1**:182–3.

Chalmers I. What do I want from health research and researchers when I am a patient? BMJ 1995;**310**:1315–1318.

Chalmers I. Evidence of the effects of health care: a plea for a single standard across 'orthodox' and 'complementary' medicine. Complementary Therapies in Medicine 1998;**6**:211–213.

Koes BW, Assendelft WJ, van der Heijen GJMG, Bouter LM, Knipschild PG. Spinal manipulation and mobilisation for back and neck pain: a blinded review. *BMJ* 1991;**303**:1298–303.

Skrabanek P. Acupuncture and the age of unreason. *Lancet* 1984;**1**:1169–1171.

Preface

Most doctors are aware of the fact that complementary and alternative medicine (CAM) is used by many of their patients. In recent years, conventional medicine has demonstrated an increased general openness towards CAM. This new attitude foremost requires knowledge about the facts. What facts? Some sceptics still insist that all CAM is mumbo jumbo steeped in belief and devoid of evidence. We predict that these people will find our book nothing short of revolutionary.

Our approach is not to reinvent the wheel but to simply apply the rules of science and evidence-based medicine to CAM. It is true, CAM used to be largely devoid of evidence—but not any longer! In the past decade alone, there have been hundreds of clinical trials and dozens of meta-analyses. Our objective is to summarize these data in an accessible, matter-of-fact fashion avoiding the sometimes obscure jargon of CAM.

Because of its current popularity, clinicians need to know what CAM is all about. It is not just embarrassing to find that our patients know more about the pros and cons of, for example, using herbal remedies to treat their menopausal symptoms. In fact, it is our ethical, moral, and legal duty to advise patients about the best treatments for any given condition—and today, this often includes CAM. This book is aimed at enabling medical students, GPs and hospital doctors to fulfill this task responsibly.

Edzard Ernst
Max H Pittler
Barbara Wider
Kate Boddy
Exeter, May 2007

* The authors of this book are not aware of any conflicts of interest, financial or otherwise.

Contents

Reviewers

With thanks to the following people for their constructive review feedback:

Mabel Aghadiuno
Helen Beaumont
Helen Burgess
Andy Chivers
Gemma Evans
Jean Simner
Ian Woollands

How to use chapters 3, 4, and 5

The complementary treatments covered in Chapters 3 and 4 are those which are popular with patients. The conditions in Chapter 5 are those which are commonly seen in primary care and frequently treated with CAM. Furthermore, evidence relating to effectiveness had to be available for the respective topics to be included.

Chapter content

Each topic consists of two parts. The first provides an overview of the treatment or condition. In the second part—the 'Clinical bottom line'—the clinical evidence for each treatment or condition is presented. This is based on systematic literature searches carried out in a number of general medical and specialist databases through to April 2007.

Evidence evaluation

The retrieved evidence was assessed for:
- Its methodological quality (i.e. the validity and reliability of the studies).
- Its level (the highest level being systematic review/meta-analysis, followed by randomized clinical trial, controlled clinical trial, and uncontrolled trial).
- Its volume (i.e. the number of studies and their sample sizes).
- Expectations of harms.

Evidence categories

Treatments or conditions were accordingly assigned to six standardized categories. These categories are the ones used by the BMJ *Clinical Evidence* as most health care professionals will be familiar with them.

Beneficial: effectiveness has been demonstrated by clear evidence from RCTs, and expectation of harms is small compared with the benefits.

Likely to be beneficial: effectiveness is less well established than for those listed under 'beneficial'.

Trade off between benefits and harms: clinicians and patients should weigh up the beneficial and harmful effects according to individual circumstances and priorities.

Unknown effectiveness: there are currently insufficient data or data of inadequate quality.

Unlikely to be beneficial: lack of effectiveness is less well established than for those listed under 'likely to be ineffective or harmful'.

Likely to be ineffective or harmful: for which ineffectiveness or harmfulness has been demonstrated by clear evidence.

It is important to note that absence of evidence of effectiveness does not imply absence of effectiveness.

Tables of systematic up-to-date reviews

Where systematic reviews of treatments were available they were summarized and included in table format. Treatments had to be beneficial or likely to be beneficial and up-to-date (i.e. recent or not contradicting evidence subsequently published) in order to be included.

Safety issues

The precautionary principle has been applied, i.e. a treatment is not considered risk-free unless evidence suggests otherwise; this is particularly pertinent to pregnancy and lactation which are cited as contraindications for all medicines. Only direct risks are listed i.e. any indirect risks such as inadequately trained practitioners, or delay of effective treatment are not included.

5 Conditions **261**

Cardiology

Dermatology

Diabetology

Gastroenterology

Abbreviations

AIDS	acquired immune deficiency syndrome
ADHD	attention deficit hyperactivity disorder
CAM	complementary and alternative medicine
COPD	chronic obstructive pulmonary disease
CVI	chronic venous insufficiency
DHA	docosahexaenoic acid
EPA	eicosapentaenoic acid
g	gram/s
GP	general practitioner
HDL	high density lipoprotein
HIV	human immunodeficiency virus
IBS	irritable bowel syndrome
L	litre
LDL	low density lipoprotein
mg	milligram/s
mcg	microgram/s
NHS	National Health Service
NSAIDs	non-steroidal anti-inflammatory drugs
RA	rheumatoid arthritis
UK	United Kingdom
UTI	urinary tract infection

Chapter 1

General issues

What is CAM?

Complementary and alternative medicine (CAM) refers to a diverse array of treatment modalities and diagnostic techniques that are not presently considered part of conventional/mainstream medicine and emphasizes a holistic approach towards health care. Although most people have a good idea which treatments are CAM and which are not, there remains some confusion about how to define CAM.

A number of terms and definitions exist (Table 1.1) which mostly define CAM by what it is not, e.g., not provided in routine health care, not taught to medical students, not scientifically proven. In the 1970s and 1980s, the term 'alternative medicine' was popular, highlighting that CAM treatment approaches are used instead of conventional or mainstream treatments, thus clearly separating the two. Later, the term 'complementary medicine' was deemed more appropriate; it describes treatments used in addition to conventional medicine, i.e. highlighting that the two systems are used in parallel. Over the years, 'complementary and alternative medicine' established itself as an umbrella term. The focus of the term shifted from mainly meaning 'outside the mainstream medical system' to describing a group of therapeutic approaches with certain similar characteristics. Nowadays 'integrated' or (American) 'integrative medicine' have become buzz words claiming to comprise 'the best of both systems' by combining conventional with CAM treatments (see 📖 Evidence-based medicine or integrative medicine).

Which therapies are CAM?

To help understand and group the many divergent CAM therapies (Table 1.2), the US National Centre for Complementary and Alternative Medicine (NCCAM) has classified CAM and created five categories[1]:

Alternative medical systems

These are complete systems of theory and practice. Examples of alternative medical systems that have developed in Western cultures include homeopathic medicine and naturopathic medicine. Examples of systems that have developed in non-Western cultures include traditional Chinese medicine and Ayurveda.

Mind-body interventions

Interventions using a variety of techniques designed to enhance the mind's capacity to affect bodily function and symptoms. Examples include meditation, prayer, mental healing, and therapies that use creative outlets such as art, music, or dance.

Biologically-based therapies

Biologically based therapies in CAM use substances found in nature, such as herbs, foods, and vitamins. Examples include dietary supplements and herbal products.

Manipulative and body-based methods

Manipulative and body-based methods in CAM are based on manipulation and/or movement of one or more parts of the body. Some examples include chiropractic or osteopathic manipulation and massage.

Energy therapies

Energy therapies involve the use of energy fields. Biofield therapies are intended to affect energy fields that purportedly surround and penetrate the human body. Examples include qigong, Reiki, and Therapeutic Touch. Bioelectromagnetic-based therapies involve the unconventional use of electromagnetic fields, such as pulsed fields or magnetic fields.

Table 1.1 Selection of currently used definitions of CAM

Definition	Source
'CAM is a group of diverse medical and health care systems, practices, and products that are not presently considered to be part of conventional medicine.'	NCCAM, USA, http://nccam.nih.gov/health/whatiscam/#1
'CAM refers to a broad set of health care practices that are not part of a country's own tradition and not integrated into the dominant health care system. Other terms sometimes used to describe these health care practices include "natural medicine", "non-conventional medicine" and "holistic medicine".'	World Health Organization. Guidelines on developing consumer information on proper use of traditional, complementary and alternative medicine. Geneva: World Health Organization;2004:xiii
'Complementary medicine refers to a group of therapeutic and diagnostic disciplines that exist largely outside the institutions where conventional health care is taught and provided.'	Zollman C, Vickers A. What is complementary medicine? *BMJ* 1999;**319**:693–6
'CAM is a broad domain of healing resources that encompasses all health systems, modalities, and practices and their accompanying theories and beliefs, other than those intrinsic to the politically dominant health systems of a particular society or culture in a given historical period.'	Cochrane Collaboration, http://www.compmed.umm.edu/Cochrane.asp
'Complementary medicine is diagnosis, treatment and/or prevention which complements mainstream medicine by contributing to a common whole, satisfying a demand not met by orthodoxy, or diversifying the conceptual framework of medicine.'	Ernst E, Resch K L, Mills S *et al.* Complementary medicine—a definition. *Br J Gen Pract* 1995;**309**:107–11

Table 1.2 Description of common CAM therapies

Therapy	Description
Acupuncture	Insertion of needles into the skin at special sites, known as points, for therapeutic or preventive purposes
Alexander technique	Psychophysical re-education to improve postural balance and coordination
Applied kinesiology	Diagnostic technique using muscle strength as an indicator to diagnose and treat illness or allergy
Aromatherapy	Use of plant essences for therapeutic purposes, usually with massage
Bach flower remedies	System that uses plant infusions to balance emotional disturbances
Chiropractic	Diagnosis, treatment and prevention of mechanical disorders of the musculoskeletal system, emphasis on manual treatments including spinal manipulation
Guided imagery	Controlled use of mental images for therapeutic purposes
Herbal medicine	Medical use of preparations made from plant material
Homeopathy	A therapeutic method, developed by Samuel Hahnemann, often using highly diluted preparations of substances whose effects when administered to healthy subjects in less diluted form correspond to the manifestations of the disorder in the unwell patient
Hypnotherapy	Induction of a trance-like state to facilitate relaxation and make use of enhanced suggestibility to effect behavioural changes and treat medical conditions
Iridology	A diagnostic technique using signs and impurities found on the iris
Magnet therapy	Permanent or pulsed magnetic fields applied to head or other parts of body
Massage	Manipulation of the soft tissues of the whole body using pressure, friction, and traction
Meditation	Diverse range of techniques based on listening to the breath, repeating a mantra, focusing attention to bring about a state of calm
Osteopathy	Manipulation of soft tissues and the mobilization/manipulation of peripheral or spinal joints
Reflexology	Manual pressure applied to specific areas of the feet (sometimes hands or ears) that are believed to correspond with other areas or organs of the body to prevent and treat illness

Table 1.2 (Contd.)

Therapy	Description
Relaxation	Various techniques for eliciting the 'relaxation response' of the autonomic nervous system
Spiritual healing	Channelling of 'healing' energy from a healer to a patient to treat an illness
Tai chi	System based on Chinese philosophy and martial arts using specific movements to enhance wellbeing
Yoga	A mind-body intervention including gentle stretching, exercises for breath control and meditation

Reference

1. What is complementary and alternative medicine? http://nccam.nih.gov/health/whatiscam (accessed 16 October, 2006).

Common misconceptions about CAM

The fact that CAM is a 'patient-driven' movement has numerous implications, one of which is that discussions about its value or otherwise are not confined to healthcare professionals or to the medical literature. In fact, it sometimes seems that most people have strong opinions about CAM, not just consumers but also journalists, politicians, etc. In turn, this phenomenon has led to an endless array of misconceptions. Here is a selection of the most common ones.

CAM is unscientific

Conventional medicine is struggling to be scientific. Yet the application of the scientific method to medicine is relatively young and not all the procedures of conventional medicine have sound scientific bases. Undoubtedly, the scientific foundations of CAM are much more shaky than those of conventional medicine. However, given the paucity of resources and the backing from the scientific community, CAM is increasingly successful in becoming scientific as much of this book demonstrates.

CAM is known to be worthless

Some CAM approaches have indeed been shown to be wrong and ineffective. Yet to generalize in the above manner is not correct. As long as a remedy has not been tested, it cannot be labelled to be either effective or ineffective. Furthermore there are many areas within CAM which have shown much promise—and this book provides ample evidence in support.

CAM is implausible

True, CAM often lacks a sound theoretical basis and tends to substitute this lack with a 'philosophy'. Philosophies, like religions, are difficult to prove right or wrong. This, however, is not to say that the remedy associated with such a philosophy is useless. The history of medicine abounds with examples of therapies that were once used on the basis of a totally false rationale. Eventually the concepts were corrected and the therapy, which, of course, had to have a certain level of effectiveness to begin with, became established for defined conditions. In other words, just because the philosophy of a CAM approach, e.g. traditional Chinese medicine, is in conflict with science, a treatment, e.g. acupuncture, is not necessarily ineffective.

CAM is no more than a placebo

The current popularity of CAM puzzles many mainstream doctors. On the assumption that CAM is of no specific use, its popularity is often said to be purely due to a powerful placebo effect. This might be true in some cases, but again one should not generalize. Several forms of CAM have specific actions, even to the extent that adverse effects may become a problem. Both their positive and negative effects render certain CAMs, e.g. herbal medicines, unlikely candidates for pure placebos.

Conventional medicine has nothing to learn from CAM

The reasons for people to consult CAM practitioners are complex and may range from disappointment with modern medicine to an inclination to mysticism. Whatever they are, they represent a serious criticism of the content and style of today's mainstream medicine. It follows that conventional medicine might have an important lesson to learn, a lesson about having time and empathy for the patient, about maximizing the placebo effect, and about taking seriously even minor complaints. In a way this boils down to 'good doctoring' or decent 'bedside manners' which, many patients feel, have got lost in our modern 'high-tech' medicine.

All that really matters is to help the patient

This is a frequent argument voiced by proponents of CAM. At first glance it is disarmingly powerful. The aim to help our patients is said to justify (almost) any means, certainly those of CAM. Particularly when dealing with conditions for which conventional medicine has not yet found a cure (and these seem to be the domain of CAM), the use of CAM is claimed to be justified—if nothing else, it provides comfort and hope. One must, however, point out that empathy and comfort should also be provided by conventional doctors. False hope can be tragically deceiving.

Freedom in therapeutic choice is important

This may be true, but the notion can only apply to effective treatments. Remedies which are not effective are strictly speaking no medicine at all. The patient has the right to be treated with the most effective treatment for the condition in question, taking into account, of course, the balance between risks, benefits, and costs. Freedom in therapeutic choice should not be confused with an arbitrary nature of choice.

CAM is natural, hence harmless

Many lay people think so, and the majority of CAM practitioners would also support this notion. However, doctors and therapists *should* know better. There is no such thing as a treatment without potential harm. CAM can be directly harmful, for instance when a herbal medicine is toxic or contaminated with a poisonous substance. Furthermore, CAM use is hazardous when it prevents a proper diagnosis or effective therapy. Like any other therapy, it is definitely dangerous when used incompetently. Lastly, it is harmful when it is needlessly wasting financial or other resources.

CAM shows its worth every day

This notion is often voiced by practitioners of CAM who regularly see their patients getting better under their very eyes. Everyone who attributes a clinical improvement solely to the therapy applied forgets other important factors that almost invariably play a role—the natural history of the disease, the regression towards the mean, and the placebo effect. Thus, experience as to the effectiveness of a given treatment can be misleading.

CAM has stood the 'test of time'

True, some remedies have been around for thousands of years. Could generations of therapists be so mistaken as to employ useless treatments for so long? The answer is YES. Take blood letting for instance, it was used for centuries as a panacea. Yet it only helps in very few diseases and most certainly has, during its history, killed more patients than it has ever helped. Moreover, the 'test of time' argument can easily be reversed—if therapy *xy* is known for such a long time, why has no-one yet come up with an acceptable proof for its effectiveness?

CAM defies scientific testing

Several claims are made to underpin this argument: 1) effects are too subtle to show up through the use of science's blunt instruments; 2) scientific medicine employs the wrong endpoints for the holistic concepts of CAM—individuals cannot be grouped because they are unique; 3) placebo-controlled trials are unethical.

Even though there is an element of truth in some of these claims, one ought to point out that conventional medicine has the same problems and that statistics are used *because* individuals react differently. There is no reason why any benefit that is real should become undetectable when a proper trial is set up in order to minimize systematic error. Even a therapy as 'individualized' as homeopathy can be tested in randomized, placebo-controlled, double-blind trials. Finally, endpoints like quality of life are frequently used in mainstream medicine, and there is no reason why CAM should reject this option.

Only CAM concerns itself with the whole individual

The (w)holistic argument tries to separate CAM from conventional medicine by a principle divide. The latter is said to be preoccupied merely with parts of an individual (i.e. an organ, a symptom, or even merely a laboratory value). CAM is claimed to see the wider perspective of the entire individual, including his/her surroundings, background, mind and spirit. Yet it is incorrect to claim that the holistic attitude is an invention of CAM. The truth is that it always has been an essential element of any (good) clinical practice.

Prevalence of CAM use

- To define requirements for the scientific investigation, education, and regulation of CAM, information on the level of use among the general population and specific patient populations is of interest.
- The definition of what precisely constitutes CAM differs considerably between countries.
- Historical developments and traditions mean that some therapies are firmly established in mainstream medicine in one country while they are classified as CAM in other countries. Examples include massage, hydrotherapy, and herbal medicine which are part of the mainstream medical system in many European countries, yet are considered CAM in others.
- Regardless of these national differences and their implications for research, there is evidence for a substantial increase in the use of, and demand for, CAM during the last decade.
- Inconsistencies abound in many surveys. However, it is possible to derive estimates and eventually outline the development of CAM over time (Table 1.3).

Table 1.3 One-year prevalence of CAM use in general population samples

Country and reference	Year of sampling	Sample n	Prevalence %
Australia	1993	Random 3004	48.5
Canada	1995	Representative 17626	15
Finland	1982	Random 1618	23
France	1985	Representative 1000	49
Germany	2002	Representative 1750	62.3
Hungary	1999	(not reported) 2357	13
Israel	2000	Representative 2505	10
Italy	1997–99	Representative 70898	15.6
Japan	2001	Random 1000	76
Singapore	2002	Matching 648	76
UK	2001	Representative 1794	28
US	2002	Representative 31044	62 (incl. prayer)

Why people use CAM

The main reasons why people use CAM are summarized in Box 1.1. The 'push' factors include dissatisfaction with conventional medicine and desperation. 'Pull' factors include compatibility between the philosophy of CAM and patients' own beliefs and the wish for more control over one's own health. Dissatisfaction with conventional care, need for personal control over treatment and philosophical congruence with own beliefs are good discriminators between CAM users and non-users[1].

Patients who turn to CAM as a last resort can be differentiated from those who embrace CAM for its compatibility with their own beliefs. The former group has similar scores to the general population on locus of control and maintains faith in the principles of conventional medicine. The other group of patients tries CAM because it matches their beliefs about health and illness. These individuals show a greater internal locus of control and scepticism about conventional medicine, as well as more commitment to CAM.

Many consumers are convinced that CAM is effective. Certain fundamental premises of most forms of CAM may contribute to its persuasive appeal[2]. One of these is the perceived association of CAM with nature. This is typified by certain terminology—natural rather than artificial, pure versus synthetic, and organic as opposed to processed. Natural is often wrongly equated with safe. Another fundamental component of CAM is vitalism. The enhancement or balancing of 'life forces', 'qi', 'psychic energy', etc. is central to many CAM therapies. Many forms of CAM have long traditions, sophisticated philosophies, or complex systems and concepts. This contributes to their credibility and authority. CAM tends to be person-centred. The language is one of unity and holism in contrast to the reductionist terminology of normative science. Human experience is the central element of CAM.

Many CAM users report a better relationship with their CAM practitioner than with their GP. CAM practitioners are perceived as friendlier and more personal, they treat the relationship more like a partnership and provide more time. As well as leading to greater satisfaction with patients, this may be one of the key factors in the success of CAM.

CAM can be a substitute in some situations and an adjunct in others. This has led to the concept of 'shopping for health'[3]. Rather than being specifically 'pushed' or 'pulled' towards CAM, patients simply perceive it as one of many treatment options and exercise their freedom of choice. The finding that CAM use is associated with higher levels of income seems to support the concept.

Cost and lack of information seem to be the most common reasons for not using CAM. Only a small percentage of patients report fear of their physician's disapproval as a barrier. Other frequently cited reasons for not starting or terminating CAM use are listed in Box 1.2.

Box 1.1 Determinants of CAM use

Push factors
- Dissatisfaction with conventional medicine:
  - ineffective treatments
  - adverse effects of treatments
  - poor communication with doctor
  - insufficient time with doctor
  - waiting lists
- Rejection of conventional medicine:
  - anti-science or anti-establishment attitude
- Desperation
- Cost of private conventional medical care

Pull factors
- Philosophical congruence:
  - spiritual dimension
  - emphasis on holism
  - active role of patient
  - intuitively acceptable concepts
  - natural treatments
- Personal control over treatment
- Good relationship with therapist:
  - on equal terms (empathy)
  - time for discussion
  - allows for emotional factors
- Accessible
- Increased wellbeing

Box 1.2 Reasons for not starting or terminating CAM

Not starting CAM
- Never considered it
- Not enough information
- Too expensive
- Satisfied with conventional treatment
- No belief in its effectiveness
- Doctor advised against it
- Religious/moral reasons
- Not available
- Too embarrassing

Terminating CAM
- Not helpful
- No longer affordable
- Experienced adverse effects
- Doctor advised against it

References

1. Astin J. Why patients use alternative medicine. Results of a national survey. *JAMA* 1998; **279**:1548–53.
2. Kaptchuk TJ, Eisenberg DM. The persuasive appeal of alternative medicine. *Ann Intern Med* 1998;**129**:1061–5.
3. Furnham A. Why do people choose and use complementary therapies? In: Ernst E, ed. *Complementary Medicine: an Objective Appraisal.* Oxford: Butterworth Heinemann, 1996.

The regulation of CAM

UK

The House of Lords' Select Committee on Science and Technology issued a report in 2000 which stated that 'there is considerable variation in the levels of professionalisation within the CAM world'.[1] Since this report there has been a move towards regulation but progress is slow as there is considerable fragmentation within the various therapeutic disciplines. For how to find a practitioner see 📖 Information resources, p. 32–35.

Osteopathy, chiropractic

The passing of the Osteopaths' Act in 1993 followed by the Chiropractors' Act in 1994 ended a situation whereby, subject to minor limitations, non-medically qualified practitioners were able to freely practise any complementary therapy.

Osteopathy and chiropractic are the only two complementary professions that, so far, have achieved statutory regulation in the UK. Similar to the General Medical Council of the medical profession, the General Osteopathic Council (GOC) and the General Chiropractic Council (GCC) are responsible for all aspects of professional regulation including ethics, disciplinary structures, and insurance regulations. The Council has the authority to remove practitioners from the register and prevent them from using the title 'chiropractor' or 'osteopath'. No-one who is not registered with the GOC or GCC may call themselves a 'chiropractor' or 'osteopath'.

Acupuncture

Acupuncture is not regulated by statute so far, although initiatives are underway. This means that, currently, anybody can call themselves an 'acupuncturist' regardless of education, training, or membership.

The British Acupuncture Council, one of three regulatory bodies of professional acupuncturists, accepts only members who have completed training that has been independently accredited by the British Acupuncture Accreditation Board (BAAB). Members must have completed at least three years' training and carry the letters MBAcC after their name.

For medical doctors practising acupuncture the regulating body is the British Medical Acupuncture Society. For physiotherapists in the UK the regulating body is the Acupuncture Association of Chartered Physiotherapists.

New legislation came into effect on 1st April 2006 in Scotland. Acupuncturists, except for medical practitioners practising acupuncture within a hospital or independent clinic, will need to have the practice premises licensed by the local authority.

Herbal medicine

Voluntary regulation exists in this area and, similar to acupuncture, initiatives for statutory regulation are underway. Currently however anyone can call themselves a herbalist and training varies greatly, ranging from low level correspondence courses to BScs.

The main regulatory body for Western medical herbalists is the National Institute for Medical Herbalists. Other bodies are the European Herbal Practitioner Association and the Register of Chinese Herbal Practitioners.

Herbal medicinal products generally fall into three categories: licensed herbal medicinal products, herbal medicinal products that are exempt from licensing, and food supplements. The British Herbal Medical Association represents companies involved in the manufacture or supply of herbal medicines, herbal practitioners, academics, pharmacists, and students of phytotherapy.

Herbal medicinal products that are sold with therapeutic claims are regulated by the Medicines and Healthcare Products Regulatory Agency (MHRA) and are required to hold a product licence. Those exempt from licensing also fall within the responsibility of the MHRA. Food supplements are controlled by the Department of Environment, Food and Rural Affairs (Defra).

Homeopathy

Two regulatory bodies exist in homeopathy. The Faculty of Homeopathy was incorporated by Act of Parliament in 1950 to train and examine medical doctors, vets, and other medical professionals, recognizable by the letters FFHom, MFHom, or LFHom after their name.

The Society of Homeopaths is the regulatory body mainly for non-medically qualified practitioners. Membership is currently not compulsory and anyone can call themselves a homeopath.

Aromatherapy

Training varies greatly for aromatherapists. Practitioners represented by the Aromatherapy Organisations Council, an umbrella body, must have trained to certain core standards.

Hypnotherapy

Doctors and dentists are represented by the British Association of Medical Hypnosis. There are many bodies for non-medically qualified practitioners. The National Council for Hypnotherapy represents over 1000 therapists and provides accredited training through approved schools.

Continental Europe

The legislative approach used to regulate access to CAM practice can vary widely between European countries. Mostly 'monopolistic' and 'tolerant' systems are represented.

Monopolistic systems, i.e. only medical professionals and auxiliaries are recognized by law to practise scientific medicine, have been adopted by, for example, Austria, France, Italy, Luxembourg, and Spain. The actual enforcement of this legislation also differs between countries.

Other countries such as Belgium, Denmark, Finland, Germany, the Netherlands, Norway, and Sweden have tolerant systems, i.e. although only the practice of scientific medicine is recognized, practitioners of various forms of alternative medicines are, at least to some extent, tolerated by law. Some procedures are, however, strictly reserved for physicians, such as surgery, obstetrics, or gynaecology.

In Germany, officially registered non-medically qualified practitioners (*Heilpraktiker*) are able to practise alongside physicians. They have a similar therapeutic repertoire as CAM practitioners in the UK. However, more emphasis is placed on diagnostic techniques and while CAM practitioners in the UK tend to specialize in one complementary therapy, *Heilpraktiker* normally use a wider range of different therapies. Furthermore, some therapies, which are considered complementary elsewhere (e.g. massage), are fully integrated into mainstream medicine and some are practised by medically qualified doctors, many of whom have received specialist training (*Arzt für Naturheilkunde*).

Harmonizing Europe

National differences on regulatory issues render the harmonization process across the European Union difficult indeed. The treaty of Rome guarantees the free movement of professionals within its legislative borders, although these issues effectively prohibit it in practice. Repeatedly there have been initiatives towards harmonization of non-medically qualified health practitioners[2], which have subsequently been rejected[3]. Currently it seems that a solution on the European level is far from being reached. New and creative approaches to these complex problems are required and awaited with some interest.

References

1. House of Lords Science and Technology Sixth Report. http://www.publications.parliament.uk/pa/ld199900/ldselect/ldsctech/123/12301.htm
2. Hege H. Das Lannoye-Papier. Alternativmedizin im Europäischen Parlament. *Dtsch Ärzteblatt* 1995; **92**:1543–4.
3. Watson R. European complementary medicine proposal watered down. *Br Med J* 1997; **314**:1641.

Teaching CAM to doctors

Most healthcare professionals are eager to learn more about CAM and the need for education is therefore great. Many medical schools have now started to include CAM in the undergraduate or postgraduate curricula.

What should be taught?

Generally speaking, medical education should enable future doctors to know the essential facts about CAM so that they can refer patients to practitioners and advise patients responsibly. It is not normally intended to teach medical students how to actually practice CAM. The 'House of Lords' Select Committee on Science and Technology' recommended that 'familiarization should prepare medical students for dealing with patients who are either accessing CAM or have an interest in doing so. This familiarization should cover the potential uses of CAM, the procedures involved, their potential benefits and their main weaknesses and dangers'.[1]

A first step could be to define a core of CAM practices for which sufficient evidence is available for responsible referral and advice. This book details many CAM interventions that might be considered for this core. CAM courses in US medical schools frequently cover the following topics: acupuncture (77%), herbal medicine (70%), relaxation therapies (66%), spirituality (64%), chiropractic (60%), homoeopathy (58%), and nutrition (51%).[2] In Europe the most commonly taught subjects are hydrotherapy, acupuncture, herbal medicine and chiropractic.[3] For all of these therapies, a body of evidence exists upon which CAM courses can be based, yet only 40% of European medical schools offer such courses.[4]

Doctors also need to learn about the national regulation of CAM providers (see 📖 The regulation of CAM p.16–19).

How should CAM be taught?

CAM is a controversial subject. When teaching medical students or young doctors, an objective, evidence-based approach seems mandatory. The existing knowledge regarding the effectiveness and safety of CAM should be presented with the least possible bias. 'Uncritical enthusiasm' and 'uninformed scepticism' may be prevalent in this area but cannot be considered constructive approaches.

An obvious problem seems to emerge: currently there appear to be more quasi-religious preachers of CAM than level-headed, well-informed experts who are able to adopt an evidence-based approach. In many instances, the adequate teaching of CAM may therefore require adequate education of the educators themselves.

Evaluation of courses

An important part of every educational program should be the evaluation of its success and failures. CAM can be no exception in this. In most instances, it seems advisable to employ the procedures and instruments that are already in use locally.

Funding

Funding of CAM education may prove to be difficult. It seems important that no vested interests are allowed to influence the contents of CAM courses. As the popularity of CAM becomes more widely acknowledged, funding of CAM courses is likely to become easier.

Conclusion

Vis-à-vis the increasing popularity of CAM, there is a growing need to teach doctors about it. If those opposed to integrating CAM into the already packed curricula are to be convinced, CAM education needs to be evidence-based, aimed at teaching openness rather than dogmatic belief systems.

References

1. House of Lords Select Committee on Science and Technology. Complementary and Alternative Medicine, 6th report, 1999-2000. London: Stationery Office, 2000. (Available at: http://www.parliament.the-stationery-office.co.uk/pa/ld199900/ldselect/ldsctech/123/12301.htm).
2. Brokaw JJ, Tunnicliff G, Raess BU, Saxon DW. The teaching of complementary and alternative medicine in US medical schools: a survey of course directors. *Acad Med* 2002; **77**:867–81.
3. Barberis L, De Toni E, Schiavone M, *et al.* Unconventional medicine teaching at the universities of the European Union. *J Altern Complement* Med 2001; **7**:337–43.
4. Varga O, Márton S, Molnár P. Status of complementary and alternative medicine in European medical schools. *Forsch Komplementärmed* 2006; **13**:41–5.

Legal and ethical aspects of CAM

The ethical principles of respect for autonomy, beneficence/non-maleficence, and justice apply to all medicine and therefore also to CAM. However, CAM differs in several respects from conventional medicine, and some of these differences can impact on ethical or legal issues.

Informed consent

In both clinical practice and research informed consent is mandatory. Patients must be informed about the chances of the proposed therapy alleviating their problem, about any risks of that treatment, about any other therapeutic options, and about the likely course of the condition should it remain untreated. In CAM, such fully informed consent is rarely provided. However, not obtaining it breaches ethical and legal requirements. CAM practitioners are required by their governing bodies to obtain consent from the doctors of any client whose condition may contraindicate them from treatment, e.g. cancer patient seeking massage treatment.

Referring patients to CAM practitioners

When doctors send patients to CAM practitioners they might *delegate*, i.e. ask another professional to provide care for which the doctor remains clinically accountable. In this case the doctor might incur legal liability for inappropriately delegating a task to someone who is not qualified to perform it. Alternatively they might *refer* them to CAM practitioners, particularly if the task goes beyond the doctor's own expertise. In this case there is far less danger of liability but CAM practitioners would be classed on a par with medical specialists.

The General Medical Council provides guidelines regarding accountability for doctors considering making a referral or delegating a patient's care: http://www.gmc-uk.org/guidance/good_medical_practice/working_with_colleagues/delegation_and_referral.asp

Conflicts of interest

In CAM conflicts of interest can relate to strong belief in the value of CAM. Such belief can be a hindrance to objectivity. Many published CAM articles, for instance, contain statements about their aim which make such conflicts obvious. Instead of conducting research to test hypotheses, CAM researchers often state that they want to 'prove' or 'demonstrate' the effectiveness of their therapies. In order to avoid bias, it is mandatory that any research project is an honest attempt to find the truth.

Funding

Money is scarce in CAM. Vis-à-vis the immense popularity of CAM, this raises the question of fairness. Since funds usually originate directly or indirectly from the consumer, one could argue that the level of CAM funding should reflect the current popularity of CAM. In view of the ethical principle of justice, this should be seen as an ethical issue and requires proper debate and transparent decision processes.

If financial support for a CAM project is obtained, this obviously has to be handled in the same transparent and ethical way as any sponsorship. Funding sources of CAM research are, however, frequently not mentioned in published CAM articles.

Approval from institutional review boards

CAM research can be methodologically complex and might extend beyond the areas of competence of institutional review boards (IRBs). Thus IRBs may face problems when trying to assess CAM protocols. In addition, many CAM researchers are concerned about the attitude of IRBs towards CAM and believe that CAM protocols are not always treated fairly by IRBs.

The current system of ethical review has been criticized for being unnecessarily bureaucratic, wasteful of time, money, energy, and paper, as well as slow and inconsistent. This situation tends to disadvantage CAM projects which often do not have the resources to cope with such adversity.

Many published CAM articles fail to mention any ethical review at all. In some countries, e.g. China, ethical review may not be obligatory or available. Countries like China are of obvious importance to CAM research, and it seems crucial that ethical standards are the same everywhere.

Rigour and validity of CAM research

Seven requirements need to be fulfilled for any clinical trial to be deemed ethical:
- Social and scientific value.
- Scientific validity.
- Fair subject selection.
- Favourable risk-benefit ratio.
- Independent review.
- Informed consent.
- Respect for potential and enrolled subjects.

This set of criteria is also applicable to CAM. Some CAM therapies may, for instance, be too implausible to merit research. Investigating such topics might therefore be unethical. Many authors have pointed out that much of CAM research is methodologically flawed, which can be regarded as unethical. Because there is little research culture and expertise in CAM, many would-be researchers are ill-equipped to cope with the high demands of the above criteria.

Ethics of CAM surveys

Currently, CAM generates more surveys than any other medical field. This raises several ethical issues. Surveys could, for instance, create unnecessary anxieties for the patient, particularly in relation to life-threatening illnesses such as cancer. Other CAM surveys may raise positive expectations which can lead to disappointment. Harm can be done by CAM surveys which are flawed or wasteful research projects.

Publication of CAM projects

The publication of research is governed by a set of guidelines which are not always followed in CAM. For instance, failure to disclose that an analysis was *post hoc* is unacceptable. Yet, in CAM articles, such disclosure seems more the exception than the rule. Conflicts of interest often remain undeclared. Dual publication of results without declaration is not acceptable, yet this practice is rife in CAM.

Dishonesty, misconduct, and fraud are serious problems in any medical research. Misrepresentation of data, for instance, might be construed as a forgivable error of minor importance in CAM, while in other areas of medical research it would be considered fraudulent. The lack of experience in research could be a risk factor for misconduct in CAM research.

Of all Medline-listed CAM journals, only very few require acknowledgement of sponsorship and conflicts of interest, and none insist on statements about informed consent. Conflicts of interest can be personal, professional, or financial; and they can be actual (do influence judgement) or potential (could affect judgement). In CAM this concept is often not being implemented.

Conclusion

The ethical and legal issues of CAM research and CAM practice are complex. In principle, they are not different from those in other areas of medicine. Because CAM differs in several respects from conventional medicine, the problems are, however, likely to vary in practice.

Cost-effectiveness of CAM

The level of use of CAM within any health service crucially depends on whether CAM is value for money. Many CAM enthusiasts are convinced that this is the case. Yet hard data are scare and often contradictory.

Systematic reviews of cost-analyses could overcome this uncertainty. Several such projects have recently become available. Table 1.4 provides details of three recent systematic reviews.[1-3] Canter indicated that, in the UK, CAM does represent an additional healthcare cost.[3] For acupuncture or spinal manipulation the cost per quality of adjusted life years (QALY) relative to usual care is between £6000 and £10,000 depending on the assumptions upon which calculations are based.[3]

Policy makers must judge whether the increases in quality of life achieved by CAM are worth the extra expenditure. Even though cost per QALY may compare favourably with other more expensive treatments, such as surgery, there is a ceiling to the incremental quality of life which can be achieved with any modality.

Cost-effectiveness studies are typically less rigorous than RCTs. For instance, they do not normally use blinding and placebo controls. The effectiveness side of the equation may therefore include a large proportion of non-specific effects. This means that some of the studies may be demonstrating not much more than the cost of a placebo response.

Collectively, these reviews emphasize two important points: we need better quality data and we should focus our research questions. Until high-quality evidence is available the question about CAM's cost-effectiveness remains unanswered.

Table 1.4 Systematic reviews of cost evaluation

First author	n	Type of studies included	Conclusion
Hulme[1]	19	Any type of cost evaluation	No conclusion regarding cost. A CAM sensitive approach is required
Thompson-Coon[2]	28	Any type of prospective economic analysis	No firm conclusions are possible
Canter[3]	4	UK cost-effectiveness studies	CAM in the UK probably represents an additional cost

References

1. Hulme C, Long AF. Square pegs and round holes? A review of economic evaluation in complementary and alternative medicine. *J Altern Complement Ther Med* 2005; **11**:179–88.
2. Thompson Coon J, Ernst E. A systematic review of the economic evaluation of complementary and alternative medicine. *Perfusion* 2005; **18**:202–14.
3. Canter PH, Thompson Coon J, Ernst E. Cost effectiveness of complementary medicine in the UK–a systematic review. *BMJ* 2005; **331**:880–1.

Research methodology in CAM

It is often argued that CAM treatments cannot be tested by the randomized clinical trial in the same way as conventional treatments because:

- The effects are too subtle to be detected.
- It was originally designed to assess other research questions and cannot assess holistic and individualized treatments.

Cause and effect

There is no reason why effects that are real should not manifest themselves in rigorous trials. Trials are designed to test for cause–effect relationships between intervention and outcome. They aim to minimize bias and error. They use large patient samples and statistical techniques because data from individual patients are too unreliable to establish causal relationships. Randomization and control groups have been shown to be valid principles to minimize bias and error irrespective of the tested intervention. If the effects are too subtle to be detected, it is unlikely that the treatment is of clinical benefit to the patient. Even research questions of, for example, highly individualized homeopathic treatments can be answered using rigorous trial designs.

Test of time?

Some CAM advocates argue that testing is not needed if a treatment has been used for a very long time, certainly longer than most of conventional medicine, because the 'test of time' has proven the treatment to be effective and safe. However, as history has shown, some treatments employed for a long time turned out to be useless or harmful when tested in clinical trials e.g. blood letting.

One of the most obvious and misleading features of the 'test of time' is the lack of a control. If controls are missing, a cause–effect relationship cannot be established, which renders this information unreliable when faced with decision making in clinical practice. In CAM, as in conventional medical practice, reliable evidence should be used; i.e. results from trials which rigorously control for the many confounding factors and biases that are potentially misleading and lead to decision errors.

Efficacy and effectiveness

Two broad categories of trials can be distinguished: efficacy or fastidious trials and effectiveness or pragmatic trials. A medical intervention tested for efficacy is:

- Studied in strictly controlled, optimal conditions (i.e. high internal validity).
- Aims to identify any specific effects due to the intervention.
- Ideally the effect size measured is a pure product of that specific effect.

However, because it was tested only in a narrowly defined setting this could mean that the findings are not applicable to the wider population. Thus, for an increase in internal validity there is a decrease in external validity in efficacy trials.

At the other end of the spectrum is the pragmatic trial which approximates 'real life' conditions. Pragmatic trials:

- Aim at quantifying the total therapeutic effect including specific effect, placebo- or context effects, effects of undeclared concomitant therapies, and social desirability.
- Often compare CAM to no treatment or add CAM to usual treatment and compare it to usual treatment alone.
- Allegedly provide more meaningful data for clinical decision making.
- Are valuable, if large enough, for testing whether a treatment is useful in reality once its efficacy has been established.

The most obvious problem with such trials is the lack of adequate control groups (often in addition to lack of control of selection bias and expectation). The reduced internal validity of such trials means that the findings can be interpreted in more than one way. Thus, the results of a pragmatic trial are unreliable to establish cause-effect relationships and in the absence of efficacy data, the results of pragmatic trials are of little value.

Evidence-based medicine or integrated medicine?

Integrated (in the US: integrative) healthcare is the new 'buzzword'. Confusingly the term has two different definitions. Firstly, it describes a healthcare system 'that selectively incorporates elements of CAM into comprehensive treatment plans…'. Secondly, it stands for 'health and healing rather than disease and treatment. It views patients as whole people with minds and spirits as well as bodies…'.[1]

Few would disagree with a whole person approach, particularly in primary care. This concept (holism), however, has always been a core principle of any good medicine. Creating new names for old concepts is confusing and counter-productive.

The other definition, i.e. incorporating elements of CAM into routine healthcare is usually based on the following logic: CAM is increasingly popular, most CAM-users are satisfied with it, CAM has to be paid for by the patients themselves and is hence largely a privilege of affluent people, to achieve equity we therefore must integrate CAM into routine healthcare. This seems well-intentioned but is it also convincing?

Affluence is not just associated with CAM use; it is also linked with increased cancer, gout, Champagne consumption, liposuction rates etc. Few would want to distribute these characteristics evenly across the population. In other words, popularity does not necessarily indicate usefulness.

Satisfaction with services is also not the same as the demonstration of efficacy. The missing link in the logic of integrated healthcare is the evidence that CAM does more good than harm. Integrating therapies with uncertain risk-benefit profiles or modalities which are pleasant but with uncertain health effects would merely render healthcare less evidence-based and more expensive.

Of course, not all CAM is ineffective or unsafe, and this book provides ample evidence to prove the point. CAM interventions that are demonstrably effective should be integrated and those that are not should not. As research into CAM is still in its infancy the area of uncertainty remains large. For many forms of CAM we simply cannot be sure about the balance of risk and benefit. Integrating those therapies that are supported by good data is not integrated healthcare but simply evidence-based medicine.

And what about patient choice? This concept is well-founded in our legal systems and, as physicians, we are just advisors trying to guide patients. Creating a new type of ideology that stands for incorporation of unproven practices into medical routine is a violation of this concept. Responsible advice has to be based on evidence, not on ideology.

In conclusion, the terms 'integrated healthcare' and its derivatives are either redundant or misleading. They are superfluous when representing holism; this concept is already a part of primary care. One could, of course, argue that this is true only in theory; in practice, primary care is certainly not always holistic. If this is so, creating a new term (i.e. integrated medicine) is hardly a solution. The strategy then must be to take appropriate measures in order to remedy the omission and render primary care more holistic. The terms are misleading when promoting the routine use of unproven treatments. The integration of well-documented CAM modalities is not integrated but evidence-based medicine.

Reference

1. Rees L, Weil A. Integrated medicine. *BMJ* 2001; **322**:119–20.

CAM information resources

Overview

The sheer amount of CAM information available can be overwhelming; a simple 'Google' search for the terms 'complementary OR alternative medicine', conducted in June 2006, generated 138,000,000 hits and this number grows on a daily basis. The types of information available can be loosely split into 4 categories:

- Information for CAM consumers/patients.
- Information for CAM practitioners.
- Information for clinicians/health care professionals.
- Information for researchers and academics.

Although the boundaries between these categories may be blurred, these groups have very different information needs and therefore the vast majority of resources that are available, primarily through the internet, may not be relevant or appropriate for a healthcare professional to use. Information available may also be misleading or even dangerous, encouraging consumers to try unproven and unsafe therapies.[1]

The following resources have been selected as they are considered to be high-quality and provide information that is in keeping with an evidence-based approach to CAM.

CAM specific literature databases and libraries

- *http://www.naturalstandard.com* Database providing evidence-based information about CAM. Covers, very extensively, herbs and supplements, complementary therapies, and specific conditions. For each database entry scientific data (with links to abstracts) and expert opinions are provided in the form of comprehensive monographs. The aim of the database is to facilitate clinical decision making.
- *http://www.naturaldatabase.com* An extensive database providing scientific monographs on a huge range of herbs and supplements. Each monograph provides information about use, dose, adverse effects, efficacy, and safety. Searchable by natural product, disease/condition, or drug name each monograph contains links to abstracts.
- *http://www.library.nhs.uk/cam* This database aims to include the best available evidence for CAM. It includes Cochrane systematic reviews, other systematic reviews, and Clinical Evidence reviews focusing on specific CAM interventions for various medical conditions. Information is organized according either to condition or CAM intervention. Each entry contains a list of relevant citations with links to the abstract. The primary aim of the database is to provide relevant information to clinicians.
- *http://www.bl.uk/collections/health/comalmed.html* British Library webpage that collates a variety of internet, database and book resources on CAM.

General databases

- *http://www.pubmed.gov* A database for primary literature, PubMed is a service of the US National Library of Medicine that includes over 16 million citations from MEDLINE and other life science journals for biomedical articles back to the 1950s. CAM is covered extensively. There is also a complementary medicine subset limits button to restrict searches purely to CAM. PubMed includes links to full text articles and other related resources.
- *http://www.interscience.wiley.com* Cochrane Library contains high-quality, independent evidence to inform healthcare decision-making. It includes reliable evidence from Cochrane and other systematic reviews, clinical trials, and more.
- *http://www.bl.uk/collections/health/amed.html* Allied and Complementary Medicine Database (AMED) is a unique bibliographic database produced by the Health Care Information Service of the British Library. It covers a selection of journals in three separate subject areas: several professions allied to medicine, complementary medicine, palliative care.
- *http://www.ovid.com* The Cumulative Index to Nursing and Allied Health Literature (CINAHL) database is the source of information for the professional literature of nursing, allied health, biomedicine, and healthcare.
- *http://www.embase.com/* EMBASE provides current and comprehensive information on drugs and pharmacology, and all other aspects of human medicine and related disciplines.

CAM journals: review

- *FACT - Focus on Alternative and Complementary Therapies*, review journal that aims to present a comprehensive overview of the latest evidence on CAM in an impartial and analytical way. www.pharmpress.com/fact

CAM journals: original research

- *Evidence-based Complementary and Alternative Medicine*, international peer reviewed journal publishing original research as well as reviews, commentaries and lecture series. http://ecam.oxfordjournals.org/
- *Complementary Therapies in Medicine*, publishes a variety of articles including original primary research, reviews and opinion pieces. http://www.intl.elsevierhealth.com/journals/ctim/
- *Complementary Therapies in Clinical Practice* (formerly *Complementary Therapies in Nursing and Midwifery*), provides papers addressing research, implementation of CAM in the clinical setting, legal and ethical concerns, therapy in practice, emergent social trends in CAM, therapy information and policy development. http://www.intl.elsevierhealth.com/journals/ctnm/
- *The Journal of Alternative and Complementary Therapies*, aimed at healthcare providers it contains original research, reviews, editorials and opinion pieces. http://www.liebertpub.com/publication.aspx?pub_id=3

- *Alternative Therapies in Health and Medicine*, contains news, original research, educational pieces and is concerned with the practical use of CAM. http://www.alternative-therapies.com
- *BMC Complementary and Alternative Medicine*, open-access electronic journal publishing original research articles in CAM healthcare interventions, with a specific emphasis on those that elucidate biological mechanisms of action. http://www.biomedcentral.com/bmccomplementalternmed/
- *Forschende Komplementärmedizin/Research in Complementary Medicine*, publishes original research aimed at bridging the gap between conventional medicine and CAM. http://content.karger.com

CAM organizations

- *http://nccam.nih.gov* The US National Center for Complementary and Alternative Medicine (NCCAM) is one of the 27 institutes and centers that make up the US National Institutes of Health. It is dedicated to disseminating authoritative information to the public and professionals about CAM. The website is a vast general resource containing scientific information about CAM modalities, conditions, herbs and supplements. Also contains details about trials being conducted by the centre and information about guidelines, policies and CAM training.
- *http://www.rccm.org.uk/* The Research Council for Complementary Medicine's website provides a variety of resources aimed at providing practitioners and patients with information about efficacy of CAM. One of the major resources is the Complementary and Alternative Medicine Evidence Online (CAMEOL) database which displays the systematic reviews available for each entry.
- *http://www.fihealth.org.uk/* The Foundation is a lobby group set up by the Prince of Wales to facilitate the development and delivery of integrated healthcare. The website contains resources for professionals interested in establishing integrated practices such as databases of training courses, guidelines and reports.
- *http://www.i-c-m.org.uk/* The Institute for Complementary Medicine is a UK umbrella organization providing information on complementary therapies for the public. Site includes a searchable database of registered complementary therapy practitioners, and details about courses and other resources.
- *http://www.bcma.co.uk* The British Complementary Medicine Association is an umbrella organization for over 60 CAM organizations/associations, schools and colleges. The website offers information about different CAM modalities, registered therapists, and training courses.

Finding a practitioner

- *http://www.nhsdirectory.org/* NHS health professionals can search for suitable practitioners using the NHS health directory, which is a searchable database of CAM practitioners.
- *http://www.complementaryalternatives.com/* The online magazine *Complementary Alternatives*, published in association with the NHS Trusts Association, also has a searchable practitioner database.

Diagnostic methods

We tend to think of CAM in terms of therapeutic interventions and forget that CAM has its own, unique diagnostic methods. A patient consulting, for example, a traditional Chinese acupuncturist or herbalist, or a chiropractor will be assessed by that therapist with diagnostic tools which are unknown in conventional medicine. Some CAM modalities are even purely or mainly diagnostic, e.g. iridology or kinesiology.

To be valid, any diagnostic tool has to fulfil a set of criteria:
- It has to be reproducible.
- It has to be sensitive.
- It has to be specific.

Many of the diagnostic methods of CAM have not been formally validated. When such studies are available, they usually fail to demonstrate validity of the method in question.

Bioresonance

Bioresonance is a method that uses an electronic device to receive electromagnetic waves emitted from the body. This is thought to provide valuable diagnostic information. The most rigorous assessments of this technique negate validity.

Chiropractic diagnostic techniques

Chiropractors use imaging and manual techniques to locate spinal malalignment. The most reliable tests of these methods indicate poor reliability and specificity.

Iridology

Iridologists identify irregularities in the iris. Referring to maps where each spot on the iris is related to inner organs, they use this information to diagnose abnormalities, weaknesses or diseases in specific organs. This method has been tested extensively and has been shown to be invalid.

Kinesiology

Kinesiology or applied kinesiology posits that weakness of certain muscle groups is indicative of organ malfunction. This method has been studied extensively and the most reliable results fail to demonstrate validity.

Kirlian photography

This technique generates photographic images that result when high frequency electrical currents are applied to the body. The reliability of this method has repeatedly been shown to be low.

Pulse diagnosis

Practitioners of traditional Chinese medicine study the qualities of the radial pulse (without being primarily interested in detecting arrhythmias or determining heart rate). Usually 12 different radial pulse qualities are palpated and related to the function of inner organs. The reliability of this method is generally poor.

- For patients and non-NHS health professionals it is best to approach the respective CAM organizations direct. Most therapies have their own organizations with lists of qualified practitioners. ▢ Chapter 3 provides website addresses of organizations or councils at the end of the respective therapy sections.

Reference

1. Ernst E, Schmidt K. 'Alternative' cancer cures via the Internet? *Br J Cancer* 2002; **87**:479–80.

Diagnostic methods

Radionics

This is an umbrella term for techniques such as dowsing, devining, pendulum diagnosis and its (most often electronic) derivatives. The few studies that are available indicate that radionics is not a valid diagnostic tool.

Reflexology

Reflexology uses maps of the sole of a human foot where certain areas relate to inner organs. Palpating these areas, it is believed, provides information about the function of inner organs. Several studies have shown this method to lack validity.

Tongue diagnosis

In traditional Chinese medicine the tongue is visually inspected for its colour, shape, texture, and structure and its condition is linked to human health. The results of scientific evaluations are inconclusive.

Vega-Test

This diagnostic test exists in numerous variations and is used by many acupuncturists and other CAM practitioners. An electronic device measures electromagnetic properties at acupuncture points, which allegedly provides information about health and the best treatments of disease. The most rigorous tests of this method fail to show validity.

Conclusion

This brief overview indicates that the diagnostic methods of CAM are either invalid or have not been adequately tested for validity. It follows that the likelihood of producing false positive or false negative results is high. With a false positive diagnosis, treatment might ensue which is unnecessary, harmful, or expensive. With false negative diagnoses, effective treatments can be delayed which, depending on the nature of the condition, may be life-threatening.

The inescapable conclusion seems to be that patients should only have CAM treatments once a conventional diagnosis has been made. Healthcare practitioners should insist that this is the case.

Further reading

Ernst E, Diagnostic methods. In: Ernst E, Pittler MH, Wider B, Boddy K, eds. *The Desktop Guide to Complementary and Alternative Medicine.* 2nd edn. Edinburgh: Mosby, 2006.

Complementary therapies

Acupuncture

Definition
Insertion of one or more needles into the skin and underlying tissues at acupuncture points for therapeutic or preventative purposes.

Concept
'Traditional' acupuncturists believe that the life force qi (pronounce /chee/) and the two opposing elements yin and yang govern health. Qi is thought to circulate in 12 meridians. The flow of qi can, according to acupuncturists, be influenced by stimulating acupuncture points along these meridians. Traditional acupuncturists make a diagnosis according to the principles of traditional Chinese medicine, treat patients on a highly individualized basis, and are convinced that most conditions are treatable by acupuncture.

'Western' acupuncturists view acupuncture as being based on neuro-physiological concepts. Their treatments tend to be less individualized and they focus on pain management.

Related techniques
Instead of needle insertion, several other methods are used for stimulating acupuncture points, e.g. electrical current (electroacupuncture), pressure (acupressure), heat (moxibustion), and laser light (laser-acupuncture).

Treatment
After taking a history and diagnostic procedures such as tongue or pulse diagnosis, acupuncturists usually insert 1–12 disposable needles, stimulate them manually, and leave them in situ for about 20 minutes. Treatments are typically repeated weekly, 6–8 times.

Clinical bottom line
Benefits

:😀: *Beneficial*
- Nausea and vomiting: after chemotherapy, surgery, or pregnancy-related.
- Neck pain: most studies show pain reduction.
- Osteoarthritis of the knee: most rigorous studies are positive.

😀 *Likely to be beneficial*
- Angina pectoris: preliminary data suggest pain reduction.
- Anxiety: preliminary data suggest a relaxation response.
- Back pain: most rigorous studies are positive.
- Dental pain: most rigorous studies are positive.
- Gastrointestinal endoscopy: reduction of discomfort.
- Oocyte retrieval: reduction of pain.
- Tennis elbow: short-term pain relief.

😐 *Unknown effectiveness*
- Alcohol dependence: trial data inconclusive.
- Alzheimer's disease: memory loss, studies have methodological limitations.

- Asthma, lung function: attack frequency, data conflicting.
- Cancer pain: data conflicting.
- Chemotherapy-induced leukopenia: studies are of poor quality.
- Chronic heart failure: not enough data available.
- Chronic obstructive pulmonary disease, dyspnoea: not enough data available.
- Correction of fetal breech presentation: data conflicting.
- Crohn's disease: not enough data available.
- Cystic fibrosis: preliminary data encouraging but scarce.
- Depression: data conflicting.
- Epilepsy: may reduce seizure frequency and duration yet not enough data available.
- Erectile dysfunction: not enough data available.
- Fertility: not enough data available.
- Fibromyalgia: pain, data conflicting.
- Hay fever, severity of symptoms: conflicting results.
- Headache, idiopathic: intensity and frequency of pain but data contradictory.
- Herpes zoster, pain: data conflicting.
- Hypertension, blood pressure control: conflicting results.
- Insomnia, sleep quality: studies have methodological limitations and results are contradictory.
- Irritable bowel syndrome: most studies are of poor quality.
- Labour induction: not enough data available.
- Labour pain: few and conflicting results.
- Loss of hearing: data scarce and contradictory.
- Menopause, symptom control: data conflicting.
- Migraine, intensity and frequency of pain: data contradictory.
- Mental alertness: not enough data available.
- Multiple sclerosis: data scarce with methodological limitations.
- Obesity: evidence not convincing, data contradictory.
- Parkinson's disease: data scarce and contradictory.
- Peripheral arterial disease, walking ability: not enough data available.
- Post-herpetic neuralgia: not enough data available.
- Premenstrual syndrome: might alleviate symptoms but studies have methodological limitations.
- Schizophrenia: studies are inconclusive.
- Shoulder pain: data are conflicting.
- Stroke, recovery during rehabilitation: data conflicting.
- Temporomandibular joint pain: data contradictory.
- Tinnitus: trial data contradictory.
- Ulcerative colitis: not enough data available.
- Urinary tract symptoms: not enough data available.
- Xerostomia: not enough data available.

😣 *Unlikely to be beneficial*
- HIV/AIDS, peripheral neuropathic pain.
- Rheumatoid arthritis: no beneficial effects on swollen, tender joints, patient's global assessment and disease activity.
- Tinnitus, symptom control.

⚡ *Likely to be ineffective or harmful*
- Drug dependence, cocaine: best evidence fails to show effectiveness.
- Smoking cessation: best evidence fails to show effectiveness.

Risks
- *Contraindications:* severe bleeding disorders (needle acupuncture), first trimester of pregnancy, epilepsy.
- *Precautions/warnings:* asepsis is mandatory, electro-acupuncture for patients with pacemakers, children.
- *Adverse effects:* drowsiness, bleeding, bruising, pain during needle insertion, aggravation of presenting symptom, pneumothorax, infections.
- *Interactions:* cardiac pacemakers.

Conclusions

- Several indications are supported by good evidence
- The risks are generally small
- For a range of conditions, the benefits of acupuncture seem to outweigh its risks

Table 3.1 Systematic up-to-date reviews where acupuncture has been found to be beneficial or likely to be beneficial

Condition	Source	No. of trials/ patients	Original conclusion
Back pain	*Ann Intern Med* 2005; **142**: 651–63	N=33/n=1673	Acupuncture effectively relieves chronic low back pain
Nausea and vomiting after chemotherapy	*Cochrane Database Syst Rev* 2006; **2**: CD002285	N=11/n=1247	Complements data on post-operative nausea and vomiting suggesting a biologic effect of acupuncture-point stimulation
Nausea and vomiting, pregnancy-related	*Explore (NY)* 2006; **2**:412–21	N=13/n=1615	Acupressure and electrical stimulation had greater impact than the acupuncture methods in the treatment of nausea and vomiting in pregnant women
Neck pain	*Spine* 2007; **2**:36–43	N=10/n=661	There is moderate evidence that acupuncture relieves pain better than some sham treatments
Osteoarthritis	*Rheumatology* 2006; **45**:1331–7	N=18/n=1891	Sham-controlled RCTs suggest specific effects of acupuncture for pain control

Further reading

Ernst E. Acupuncture–a critical analysis. *J Intern Med* 2006: **259**:125–37.
Hepen CH, Wortman Chow V. *Pocket Atlas of Acupuncture*. Stuttgart: Thieme, 2006.
British Acupuncture Council. http://www.acupuncture.org.uk/

Alexander technique

Definition

Psychophysical re-education for improving posture and co-ordination based on correcting the relationship between head, neck, and spine during activity. Developed by the Australian actor Frederick M. Alexander at the end of the 19th century.

Concept

The method is based on three principles: 1) function is affected by use; 2) an organism functions as a whole; 3) the position of the head, neck, and spine are important for the body to function well.

Related techniques

Physiotherapy, Feldenkrais, rolfing, Tragerwork, yoga.

Treatment

A teacher guides the patient through a complex series of one-to-one lessons using a gentle hands-on approach to teach movement with the head leading and the spine following. Each session lasts about one hour. Regular (life-long) home treatment is advised. After 30 lessons the patient is able to carry on independently. Specialized courses and refresher lessons are available.

Clinical bottom line

Benefits

😕 *Unknown effectiveness*

- Asthma: not enough data available.
- Back pain: not enough data available.
- Parkinson's disease, disability: not enough data available.

Risks

- *Contraindications:* none known.
- *Precautions/warnings:* none known.
- *Adverse effects:* none known.
- *Interactions:* none known.

Conclusions

- Alexander technique has not convincingly been shown to be effective for any indication
- No serious risks are on record
- A risk–benefit balance fails to be positive

Further reading

Ernst E, Canter PH. The Alexander technique: a systematic review of controlled clinical trials. *Forsch Komplementarmed Klass Naturheilkd* 2003: **10**:325–9.
The Society of Teachers of The Alexander Technique. http://www.stat.org.uk/

Applied kinesiology

Definition
Method of testing the strength of groups of muscles to diagnose and treat illness. The technique was developed by George Goodheart in the 1960s.

Concept
Practitioners assume that specific health problems are associated with weaknesses of specific groups of muscles. They use manual techniques to identify these groups and to test the adequacy of specific treatments (e.g. homeopathic remedies).

Related techniques
Conventional tests of muscular function.

Treatment
The therapist takes a medical history and conducts muscle testing to diagnose illness or predispositions for disease. Subsequently practitioners identify the optimal therapy (e.g. a homeopathic remedy) via similar manual testing. One session may last for about 30 minutes and several (6–10) repeat sessions may be required.

Clinical bottom line
Benefits
🔯 *Likely to be ineffective or harmful*
- Several studies have shown this test to be not valid for diagnosing medical conditions. It can therefore not be accepted as a reliable basis for diagnosis or treatment of any medical condition.

Risks
- *Contraindications:* none known.
- *Precautions/warnings:* none known.
- *Adverse effects:* false positive or false negative diagnoses may represent a serious risk to human health.
- *Interactions:* none known.

Conclusions
- Validity has been refuted in several investigations
- Risk of false positive or false negative diagnoses
- Risk–benefit balance fails to be positive

Further reading
Frost R. Applied Kinesiology: *A Training Manual and Reference Book of Basic Principles.* Berkely, CA: North Atlantic Books, 2002.

Aromatherapy

Definition
The medicinal use of plant essences.

Concept
The fact that scents activate the olfactory sense and thus affect the brain is undisputed. Some oils may be absorbed through the skin. The largely open question is whether these effects lead to specific health benefits.

Related techniques
Massage, inhalation, topical treatments.

Treatment
Usually diluted essential (from essence) oils are applied through gentle massage. The individual choice of oil is determined through the experience of the therapist. Occasionally, essential oils are also used in baths or diffusers. One session typically lasts around 1 hour. A full series may include about 10 sessions.

Clinical bottom line
Benefits

☼ *Beneficial*
- Cancer palliation: aromatherapy improves quality of life.

☻ *Likely to be beneficial*
- Anxiety: most data indicate a positive effect.
- Back pain: most trials suggest pain relief.

☻ *Unknown effectiveness*
- Acne: tea tree oil, antimicrobial action but evidence is inconclusive.
- Alopecia areata: not enough data available.
- Alzheimer's disease, symptom control: wellbeing but not enough data available.
- Arthritis pain: not enough data available.
- Bronchitis prevention: not enough data available.
- Constipation: not enough data available.
- Dementia, agitation: not enough data available.
- Depression: not enough data available.
- Dysmenorrhoea: not enough data available.
- Fungal infection: tea tree oil, evidence is conflicting.
- Hair loss: preliminary data suggest positive effects but not enough data available.
- Insomnia: not enough data available.
- Labour pain: data for pain relief scarce and methodologically limited.
- Postnatal perineal discomfort: not enough data available.
- Postoperative nausea: not enough data available.
- Pruritus of haemodialysis patients: not enough data available.

�֎ *Likely to be ineffective or harmful*
- Cancer pain: not effective for symptom control.

Risks
- *Contraindications:* contagious disease, pregnancy, epilepsy, venous thrombosis, varicose veins, broken skin, recent surgery, circulatory disorders.
- *Precautions/warnings:* essential undiluted oils should not be taken orally, photosensitivity, some oils may be carcinogenic.
- *Adverse effects:* allergic reactions, phototoxicity, nausea, headache.
- *Interactions:* depending on the specific pharmacological actions (if any) of the essential oil.

Conclusions

- May improve quality of life in cancer palliation and is likely to have a positive effect on anxiety and back pain; no compelling evidence exists for any other indication
- Few serious risks are on record
- As an adjunctive therapy for improving quality of life of cancer patients, the risk–benefit balance is positive, it is likely positive for anxiety and back pain

Table 3.2 Systematic up-to-date review where aromatherapy has been found to be beneficial or likely to be beneficial

Condition	Source	No. of trials/ patients	Original conclusion
Cancer palliation	*Cochrane Database Syst Rev* 2004; **3**: CD002287	N=8/n=357	Aromatherapy generates short-term benefits on psychological wellbeing

Further reading

Lis-Balchin M. *Aromatherapy Science: a Guide for Healthcare Professionals.* London: Pharmaceutical Press, 2006.
The Aromatherapy Council. http://www.aromatherapycouncil.co.uk/

Autogenic training

Definition

An autosuggestive technique developed in the early 20th century by Johannes Schulz aimed at teaching individuals to 'switch off' the stress response at will.

Concept

Autogenic training produces profound relaxation and a near-hypnotic state. It is assumed that this controls psychoemotional stress which, in turn, has positive health effects.

Related techniques

Relaxation, self-hypnosis, meditation.

Treatment

Autogenic training is usually taught in groups. The participants learn simple auto-suggestive exercises, e.g. feeling warmth in their hands and feet. This progresses to more complex tasks. The technique is first learnt in about a dozen group sessions, subsequently it should be practised regularly without supervision.

Clinical bottom line

Benefits

☺ *Likely to be beneficial*

- Depression: encouraging results as adjunctive therapy.
- Insomnia: although data methodologically limited they suggest an improvement of sleep.
- Hypertension: although studies methodologically limited, overall they suggest a positive effect.

☹ *Unknown effectiveness*

- Anxiety: studies methodologically limited.
- Asthma: studies contradictory.
- Eczema, control of itching: not enough data available.
- Headache: not superior to other interventions in terms of symptom control, data have methodological limitations.
- Pain: only few studies available, most of which are methodologically limited.

Risks

- *Contraindications:* psychoses.
- *Precautions/warnings:* psychoses.
- *Adverse effects:* none known.
- *Interactions:* none known.

Conclusions

- There is encouraging evidence that autogenic training might be a useful adjunctive therapy for depression, insomnia, and hypertension
- Good safety record
- Risk–benefit balance is likely to be positive for depression, insomnia and hypertension

Further reading

Kermani K. *Autogenic Training: The Effective Holistic Way to Better Health.* London: Souvenir Press 1996.
The British Autogenic Society. http://www.autogenic-therapy.org.uk/

Ayurveda

Definition
Ancient Indian philosophy which forms the basis of a traditional medical system.

Concept
In Ayurveda, it is assumed that humans are characterized by their unique composition of three 'doshas' or metabolic types: Vata, Pitta, Kapha. Imbalance of the doshas results in illness and can be restored by Ayurvedic treatments, which may include herbal remedies, psychological approaches, detoxification procedures, relaxation techniques, and physical exercises and accounts for the biologic individuality of the patient.

Related techniques
Diet, herbal medicine, massage, meditation, yoga.

Treatment
The practitioner takes a medical history, conducts a physical examination (including perhaps tongue diagnosis) and prescribes an individualized set of treatments. Treatment is usually long-term, particularly for chronic conditions. It may also include preventative measures.

Clinical bottom line
Benefit
- No controlled clinical trials are available testing the entire 'package' of Ayurvedic medicine. Studies are usually focused on single modalities, e.g. yoga, herbs, meditation. The evidence relating to these treatments is dealt with in other chapters in this book.

Risks
- *Contraindications:* see specific modality.
- *Precautions/warnings:* see specific modality.
- *Adverse effects:* see specific modality.
- *Interactions:* see specific modality.

Conclusions
- No trial data on Ayurveda as a whole system is available
- Depending on the specific modalities used, the risks can be considerable, e.g. heavy metal contamination from Ayurvedic medicines
- The risk–benefit balance fails to be positive

Further reading
Mishra LC (Ed). *Scientific Basis for Ayurvedic Therapies.* Boca Raton: CRC Press, 2004.

(Bach) Flower Remedies

Definition
A therapeutic system that employs specially prepared plant infusions to balance physical and emotional disturbances. It was developed by Edward Bach (1886–1936), a microbiologist at the Royal London Homeopathic Hospital, about 100 years ago.

Concept
Therapists believe that all human illness is rooted in emotional imbalances. Bach discovered 38 remedies, each of which is thought to normalize specific imbalances. The remedies are produced by placing freshly picked flowers into spring water, into which brandy is later added for the purpose of preservation. Therapists prescribe highly individualized remedies that are based on the emotional imbalances of the patient in question.

Related techniques
Homeopathy (also highly diluted remedies).

Treatment
Often remedies are self-prescribed and bought over the counter. If patients consult a specialized therapist, a detailed history will be taken, little emphasis is placed on physical examinations and the individualized remedy is prescribed. Depending on the nature of the condition one prescription may suffice or, for persistent problems, remedies are taken long-term.

Clinical bottom line
Benefits
✖ Likely to be ineffective or harmful
- Anxiety: best studies fail to show an effect.
- Attention deficit disorder: likely to be ineffective.
- Stress: Rescue Remedy, data show no specific effects.

Risks
- Contraindications: none known.
- Precautions/warnings: none known.
- Adverse effects: none known.
- Interactions: none known.

Conclusions
- No evidence of effectiveness for any condition
- No serious safety issues
- The risk–benefit balance fails to be positive

Further reading
Bach E. Bach Flower Remedies. Chicago: Keats Publishing, 1997.

Biofeedback

Definition
The use of instrumentation to monitor, amplify, and feed back information on physiological responses so that a patient can learn to regulate these responses. Many experts would categorize biofeedback as a conventional treatment.

Concept
Patients are trained to learn to control involuntary bodily functions like brain activity, heart rate, or muscle activity. In order to achieve this goal, the function (e.g. heart rate) is made visible or audible. Gaining control over the function is claimed to result in health gains via a relaxation response.

Related techniques
Other mind–body therapies such as hypnotherapy or autogenic training.

Treatment
Practitioners of biofeedback normally practice a range of therapies. The initial consultation may include a medical history and examination to ascertain that biofeedback is indicated. The initial session may last about 1 hour. Subsequent sessions may be slightly shorter. The patient is familiarized with the technical equipment and taught how to gain control over the signals they receive, e.g. heart rate or muscular activity. Biofeedback is rarely used as a sole treatment but usually as an adjunct to other treatments. Depending on the chronicity of the condition, treatments may continue weekly for 2–3 months. Sometimes long-term home therapy is possible.

Clinical bottom line
Benefits
☺ *Beneficial*
- Faecal incontinence: bowel control.
- Headache: pain intensity.
- Hypertension: blood pressure control.
- Migraine: reduction of attack frequency.
- Urinary stress incontinence: bladder control.

☺ *Likely to be beneficial*
- Alcohol dependence: control over drinking.
- Anismus: pain reduction.
- Asthma: might improve symptoms or reduce need for medication.
- Constipation: increase of stool frequency.
- Headache, severity/frequency: data are not uniformly positive.
- Raynaud's phenomenon: thermal feedback reduces severity and frequency of attacks.

☺ *Unknown effectiveness*
- Anxiety: data contradictory.
- Back pain: not enough data available.

- Chronic obstructive pulmonary disease, dyspnoea: data conflicting.
- Chronic pain: data conflicting.
- Crohn's disease, symptom control: not enough data available.
- Diabetes type II, metabolic control: not enough data available.
- Eczema, itch, severity of skin lesions: not enough data available.
- Epilepsy, EEG biofeedback: not enough data available.
- Erectile dysfunction: data has methodological limitations.
- Fibromyalgia, pain: data has methodological limitations.
- Insomnia: sleep latency, data conflicting.
- Labour pain: data for pain relief conflicting.
- Patello femoral pain: not enough data available.
- Peripheral arterial occlusive disease, walking ability/pain: not enough data available.
- Premenstrual syndrome, symptom control: not enough data available.
- Prostatitis, chronic: pain, not enough data available.
- Stress management: data conflicting.
- Stroke rehabilitation, mobility: but not enough data available.
- Temporomandibular pain: not enough data available.
- Tinnitus, symptom control: data are scarce, methodologically limited and conflicting.
- Ulcerative colitis, symptom control: not enough data available.
- Vulvar vestibulitis: not enough data available.

😕 *Unlikely to be beneficial*
- Irritable bowel syndrome: as part of a multi-component treatment no effects on overall symptom scores.

💀 *Likely to be ineffective or harmful*
- Nausea/vomiting, chemotherapy-induced, motion sickness, severity/frequency: not effective compared to relaxation therapy.

Risks
- *Contraindications:* psychiatric illness.
- *Precautions/warnings:* medications acting on the psyche.
- *Adverse effects:* anxiety, dizziness, disorientation.
- *Interactions:* drugs acting on the same body function.

Conclusions

- Effectiveness for several indications is supported by sound data
- Encouraging safety record
- Risk–benefit balance is positive for several conditions

Table 3.3 Systematic up-to-date reviews where biofeedback has been found to be beneficial or likely to be beneficial

Condition	Source	No. of trials/ patients	Original conclusion
Headache	*Cephalalgia* 2006; **26**:1411–26	N=23/n=935	Treatments lead to improvement (up to 1 year) in headache status
Migraine	*Pain* 2007; **128**: 111–27	N=55/n=2229	A medium effect size of 0.58 resulted for all biofeedback interventions
Raynaud's phenomenon	*Appl Psychophsiol Biofeedback* 2006; **31**:203–16	N=3/n=not available	RCTs demonstrate superiority or equivalence to control conditions
Urinary incontinence	*Appl Psychophsiol Biofeedback* 2006; **31**:187–201	N=28/n=not available	Overall mean improvement was 73%

Further reading

Schwartz MS, Andrasik F. *Biofeedback: A Practitioner's Guide*. New York: Guilford Press, 2005.

Chelation therapy

Definition
Chelation therapy involves the intravenous infusion of ethylene diamine tetraacetic acid (EDTA). In CAM it is used in the hope that this removes minerals, toxins, or metabolic waste from the blood.

Concept
Originally proponents believed that chelation would remove calcium deposits from the arterial wall and thus revise arteriosclerotic changes. When this theory became untenable it was postulated that chelation works as an antioxidant or reduces reperfusion injury or has haemor-rheological effects.

Related techniques
In conventional medicine chelation therapy is used for heavy metal poisoning for which it is highly effective.

Treatment
After a conventional medical history and diagnostic procedures, patients are given the infusion during 1–3 hours, usually in the supine position. EDTA is a powerful chelating agent which eliminates minerals and other essential substances from the blood stream. Thus therapists often supplement vitamins, trace elements, and iron, during therapy or afterwards. A full series of treatments can consist of 10–30 sessions.

Clinical bottom line
Benefits

🔯 *Likely to be ineffective or harmful*
- Likely to be ineffective for arteriosclerotic diseases such as peripheral arterial occlusive disease or coronary heart disease.

Risks
- *Contraindications:* unstable coronary heart disease, aneurysms.
- *Precautions/warnings:* renal insufficiency, pregnancy, bleeding abnormality, surgery within the last 24 hours.
- *Adverse effects:* serious adverse effects include renal failure, arrhythmias, tetany, hypoglycaemia, hypotension, haematoma, convulsions, respiratory arrest.
- *Interactions:* affects the renal clearance of drugs.

Conclusions
- Efficacy of chelation therapy as used in CAM is unlikely
- It is associated with considerable risks
- Chelation therapy as used in CAM does not have a positive risk–benefit balance

Further reading

Cranton EM. *A Textbook on EDTA Chelation Therapy*. Charlottesville, VA: Hampton Roads Publishing, 2001.

Seely DM, Wu P, Mills EJ. EDTA chelation therapy for cardiovascular disease: a systematic review. *BMC Cardiovasc Disord* 2005; **5**:32.

Chiropractic

Definition

Chiropractic is a form of healthcare founded by DD Palmer (1845–1913) that focuses on the relationship between the body's structure, primarily the spine, and function. Chiropractors frequently use vertebral manipulation.

Concept

Initially chiropractors believed that 'subluxations' of the vertebrae cause illness by blocking the flow of a 'vital force' (innate intelligence). Chiropractic was thought to be a panacea. Today these concepts have been modified but the notion that 'subluxation' somehow affects human health is still upheld. Chiropractors now treat mainly musculoskeletal problems.

Related techniques

Manual therapy, osteopathy, physiotherapy.

Treatment

Chiropractors normally take a medical history and conduct a thorough investigation of the spine trying to identify blockages or 'subluxations'. Subsequently these are treated with a range of manipulative techniques supplemented by lifestyle advice etc. One session typically lasts about 30 minutes. A series of treatments may consist of 12 or more sessions. Chronic conditions may require more treatments. Many chiropractors recommend regular 'maintenance' therapy i.e. prophylactic treatment for apparently healthy people.

Clinical bottom line

Benefits

☺ *Likely to be beneficial*

- Back pain: spinal manipulation is superior to demonstrably harmful treatments in this condition (e.g. bed rest) or to sham manipulation but not more effective than conventional options (e.g. exercise).

☻ *Unknown effectiveness*

- Angina pectoris: not enough data available.
- Headache, frequency/severity of pain: studies conflicting.
- Migraine, frequency/severity of pain: studies conflicting.
- Infantile colic, pain: not enough data available.
- Premenstrual syndrome, symptom control: few studies available.
- Whiplash injury: not enough data available.

☹ *Unlikely to be beneficial*

- Asthma: symptom relief.
- Hypertension: blood pressure control.

☒ *Likely to be ineffective or harmful:*

- Anxiety: likely to be ineffective.
- Dysmenorrhoea: best evidence suggest ineffectiveness.
- Neck pain: spinal manipulation alone is not effective.

Risks
- *Contraindications:* osteoporosis, bleeding disorders, inflammatory, or malignant diseases of the spine.
- *Precautions/warnings:* patients with arteriosclerotic diseases of vertebral arteries.
- *Adverse effects:* about 50% of all patients experience mild adverse effects. Serious complications can be caused by cervical manipulations e.g. stroke (incidence unknown) and death due to arterial dissection.
- *Interactions:* none known.

Conclusions

- For back pain, chiropractic spinal manipulation is probably effective but not superior to exercise therapy
- Serious risks exist especially for cervical manipulation which chiropractors may perform even if the patient suffers from back pain
- The risk–benefit balance may be marginally positive for back pain, for all other conditions it is not

Table 3.4 Systematic up-to-date review where chiropractic has been found likely to be beneficial

Condition	Source	No. of trials/ patients	Original conclusion
Back pain	*Cochrane Database Syst Revs* 2004;**1**: CD000447	N=39/n=5486	There is evidence that spinal manipulation therapy is superior to other treatments

Further reading

Coulter ID. *Chiropratic. A Philosophy for Alternative Health Care.* Oxford: Butterworth Heinemann, 1999.

The General Chiropractic Council. http://www.gcc-uk.org/

Craniosacral therapy

Definition
A subtle form of hands-on treatment which is tissue-, fluid-, membrane-, and energy-oriented and very gentle in its application. Developed by the Americans William G. Southerland and John E. Upledger.

Concept
Craniosacral therapy is based on the premise that micro-rhythmic motions present in the body play an important role for health. Emphasis is placed upon alleged rhythmic motion of tissues and fluids such as cerebrospinal fluid, the intracranial and intraspinal dural membranes, cranial bones, and the sacrum. The unrestricted motion of these rhythms is believed to be important for the self-healing capabilities of the body. Treatment is based upon the use of light touch to facilitate natural motion.

Related techniques
Osteopathy.

Treatment
The initial diagnostic session is conducted by a craniosacral therapist in order to evaluate the problem. The procedure mainly involves lightly touching the skull and/or the sacrum although the location of treatment is largely determined by physiological requirements of the patient. The first session may take about 1 hour. Subsequent therapeutic sessions are often shorter. The number of sessions required is variable and depends on the nature and severity of the condition(s) treated.

Clinical bottom line
Benefits
☹ *Unknown effectiveness*
- There is insufficient evidence to support the effectiveness of craniosacral therapy in any condition.

Risks
- *Contraindications:* intracranial aneurysm, cerebral haemorrhage, subdural or subarachnoid bleeding, increased intracranial pressure, recent skull fractures.
- *Precautions/warnings:* none known.
- *Adverse effects:* some undesired effects reported in patients with traumatic brain syndrome; temporary worsening of symptoms and mild discomfort may occur.

Conclusions
- There is no convincing evidence for the effectiveness of craniosacral therapy for any disease or symptom
- Several risks have been associated with craniosacral therapy
- The risk–benefit balance fails to be positive

Further reading

Chaitow L. *Cranial Manipulation: Theory and Practice.* Oxford: Elsevier Churchill Livingstone, 2005.
The UK Organisation for Cranial Osteopathy. http://www.cranial.org.uk/

Feldenkrais

Definition
A treatment developed by the physicist Moshe Feldenkrais (1904–84) based on the belief that correction of posture and habitual movements can improve a range of health problems.

Concept
'Behaviour is acquired and has nothing permanent about it but our belief that it is so', stated Feldenkrais. Guided exploration of movement is thought to promote attention and awareness and improve the ability of perceptual discrimination.

Related techniques
Physiotherapy, Alexander technique.

Treatment
The therapist initially teaches 'awareness through movement' where special attention is given to the motion of the body and its parts in every-day activities. 'Functional integration', the next step, is aimed at developing optimally efficient movements under the guidance of the practitioner. Each session lasts about one hour and many sessions (including refresher courses) are required before the patient is able to practise independently at home.

Clinical bottom line
Benefits
☹ *Unknown effectiveness*
• Back pain: not enough data available.
• Eating disorder, contentment with body image: not enough data available.
• Fibromyalgia, pain: not enough data available.
• Multiple sclerosis: might reduce stress and anxiety but not enough data available.
• Neck pain: not enough data available.
• Shoulder pain: not enough data available.

Risks
• *Contraindications:* acute injuries.
• *Precautions/warnings:* disabling conditions.
• *Adverse effects:* none known.
• *Interactions:* none known.

Conclusions
• No sound evidence for effectiveness in any condition
• Good safety record
• Risk–benefit analysis fails to be positive

Further reading

Jain S, Janssen K, DeCelle S. Alexander technique and Feldenkrais method: a critical overview. *Phys Med Rehabil Clin N Am* 2004; **15**:811–25.

The Feldenkrais Guild UK. http://www.feldenkrais.co.uk/

Herbalism

Definition
The medicinal use of preparations that contain exclusively plant material.

Concept
Plants have been used since antiquity for medicinal purposes and form the origin of much of modern medicine. Modern Western herbalism or phytomedicine as practised in many European countries (e.g. Germany) is integrated into conventional medicine with compulsory education and training for physicians and pharmacists. Herbal extracts contain plant material with pharmacologically active constituents. The active principle(s) of the extract, which is in many cases unknown, may exert its effects on the molecular level and may have, for instance, enzyme-inhibiting effects (e.g. escin). A single main constituent may be active or, a complex mixture of compounds produces a combined effect. Known active constituents or marker substances may be used to standardize preparations. Other more traditional systems include Chinese herbal medicine (which is based on the concepts of yin and yang and qi energy), Ayurveda (traditional Indian medicine), and kampo (Japanese adaptation of TCM).

Synonyms/subcategories
Ayurveda, botanical medicine, herbalism, traditional Chinese herbalism, Western herbalism, kampo, phytomedicine, phytotherapy.

Treatment
During an initial treatment session the practitioner will usually take the patient's medical history to get an overall impression of the medical status and to screen for contraindications. The traditional systems may also seek information on the patient's personality and background, which may influence the selection of herbs. Individualized combinations of herbs may be prescribed. Follow-up appointments are arranged as necessary and herbal preparations and regimen reviewed and changed if appropriate. The regimen depends largely on the nature and severity of the condition, but consists generally of 1–2 appointments per week for a treatment period ranging from one to several weeks. Consultations and treatment as practised on the European continent generally follow the principles of a conventional medical appointment.

Clinical bottom line
The clinical evidence has to be evaluated according to each individual herbal preparation (□ see Chapter 4) or traditional approach. There is clinical evidence from Cochrane and other reviews for the effectiveness of a number of herbal preparations for treating various conditions (□ see Chapter 4). Traditional Chinese herbal mixtures have also been assessed in Cochrane reviews. Little evidence from systematic reviews is available for the effectiveness of other traditional herbal medical systems. Safety has been assessed in systematic reviews in relation to, for instance, individual herbs, organ systems or mechanism.

Risks

- *Contraindications:* vary for each individual herbal preparation
  (📖 see Chapter 4) but usually include pregnancy and lactation.
- *Precautions/warnings:* vary for each individual herbal preparation
  (📖 see Chapter 4).
- *Adverse effects:* plant extracts may have powerful pharmacological
  effects and therefore the risk of adverse effects is probably greater
  than with most other complementary therapies (📖 see Chapter 4).
- *Interactions:* possible interactions between different herbal preparations
  or with conventional drugs should generally be assumed and relevant
  patients should be closely monitored. Patients should be asked about
  self-prescription drug use.

Conclusions

- The most convincing evidence that exists in the area of CAM
  probably relates to a number of herbal extracts, suggesting
  effectiveness for various conditions (📖 see Chapter 4 for
  individual herbs)
- The possibility of adverse effects and interactions has to be
  considered for each herb
- The risk–benefit ratio has to be assessed for each herbal preparation
  individually (📖 see Chapter 4). A number of conditions exist for
  which conventional medical treatment is not satisfactory and
  herbalism may be a possible option

Further reading

Basch EM, Ulbricht CE (eds). *Herb and Supplement Handbook: The Clinical Bottom Line.* St Louis, MO: Elsevier Mosby, 2005.

Braun L, Cohen M. *Herbs and Natural Supplements: An Evidence-based Guide.* Sydney: Elsevier Mosby, 2005.

Capasso F, Gaginella TS, Grandolini G, Izzo AA. *Phytotherapy: A Quick Reference to Herbal Medicine.* Berlin: Springer, 2003.

The British Herbal Medicine Association. http://www.bhma.info/

Homeopathy

Definition
A therapeutic method, developed by Samuel Hahnemann (1755–1843), often using highly diluted preparations of substances whose effects when administered to healthy subjects in less diluted form correspond to the manifestations of the disorder (symptoms, clinical signs, and pathological states) in the unwell patient.

Concept
The two main axioms of homeopathy are the 'like cures like' principle (a remedy which causes a certain symptom in healthy people can be used to treat such symptoms in patients) and the notion that, by serial dilution and succussion (i.e. potentiation) a remedy does not get less but more effective.

Related techniques
Autoisopathy, Bach flower therapy, homotoxicology, isopathy, tautopathy.

Treatment
The hallmark of a homeopathic consultation is the elaborate and often extensive history taking. Most homeopaths put little emphasis upon physical examination. The skill of the homeopath is subsequently to find the remedy ('simillium') that best fits the overall picture presented by the patient. A first consultation may last for 1 hour or longer. Homeopaths need to readjust their prescriptions as the condition changes. Usually weekly consultations are required. In particular, chronic conditions may require treatments which last for many months or years.

Clinical bottom line
Benefits

😃 *Likely to be beneficial*
- Chronic fatigue syndrome: symptom control, few studies available.

😐 *Unknown effectiveness*
- AIDS, palliation: not enough data available.
- Angina pectoris: not enough data available.
- Attention deficit hyperactivity disorder: results contradictory.
- Childhood diarrhoea: data conflicting.
- Cancer palliation: data scarce and methodologically limited.
- Diarrhoea, children: not enough data available.
- Depression: lack of high quality studies.
- Fibromyalgia, pain: not enough data available.
- Loss of hearing: not enough data available.
- Osteoarthritis, pain: not enough data available.
- Overweight: not enough data available.
- Premenstrual syndrome, symptom control: not enough data available.
- Psoriasis: preliminary data available for a *Mahonia aquifolium* product which need replication.
- Rheumatoid arthritis: conflicting data for pain management.

- Seasonal allergic rhinitis, symptom control: trial data encouraging but not convincing.
- Upper respiratory tract infection, symptom control: conflicting data.

😕 *Unlikely to be beneficial*
- Anxiety: symptom control.
- Asthma: attack frequency, lung function.
- Migraine: frequency/severity of pain.

🔀 *Likely to be ineffective or harmful*
- Cancer palliation, symptom control, wellbeing.
- Headache: likely to be ineffective.
- Hypertension: likely to be ineffective.
- Labour: no effects on cervical ripening or induction of labour.
- Malaria: homeopathic vaccinations are likely to be ineffective.
- Otitis media: the most reliable trials fail to demonstrate effectiveness.
- Stroke: likely to be ineffective.
- Tinnitus: likely to be ineffective.

Risks

- *Contraindications:* none known.
- *Precautions/warnings:* none known.
- *Adverse effects:* highly dilute remedies beyond Avogadro's number cannot cause pharmacological adverse effects. Homeopaths claim that about 20% of patients experience 'homeopathic aggravations', i.e. an exacerbation of the presenting symptom caused by administering the optimal remedy.
- *Interactions:* none known.

Conclusions

- The evidence of effectiveness is encouraging for chronic fatigue syndrome
- Good safety record
- For the chronic fatigue syndrome the risk–benefit balance may be positive

Further reading

British Homeopathic Society. http://www.trusthomeopathy.org/
Walach H, Jonas WB, Ives J et al. Research on homeopathy: state of the art. *J Altern Complement Med* 2005; **11**:813–29.

Hydro-/balneotherapy

Definition
External application of water in any form or temperature (hot, cold, steam, liquid, ice). A number of variations are used, such as foot or lower leg baths, wraps, and rising temperature baths. In contrast to hydrotherapy, which generally employs normal tap water, balneotherapy is defined as baths using thermal mineral waters of at least 20°C temperature and a mineral content of at least 1g/L water from natural springs.

Concept
Hydrotherapy and balneotherapy are used particularly in continental European countries. In countries such as the UK or the US these treatments are regarded as complementary. Hydrotherapy and balneotherapy work mainly through physical (temperature, viscosity, pressure, buoyancy) and chemical (mineral content) stimuli and affect the whole body mainly via the skin. This leads to adaptation processes on the level of the vascular, muscular and metabolic systems.

Related techniques
Kneipp therapy, spa therapy, thalasso therapy.

Treatment
The treatment plan will vary according to the diagnosed condition and the treatment of a particular condition may vary between practitioners. Follow-up appointments are arranged as necessary and medicines and regimens reviewed and changed as appropriate. Depending largely on the nature and severity of the condition, the course of treatment includes generally 1–2 appointments per week for a treatment period ranging from one to several weeks.

Clinical bottom line
Benefits

😊 *Likely to be beneficial*
- Chronic venous insufficiency: cold water alone or in combination with warm water application.
- Low back pain: reduction of chronic pain through spa therapy and balneotherapy.
- Rheumatoid arthritis: seems to alleviate pain and improve quality of life.

😐 *Unknown effectiveness*
- Ankylosing spondylitis: may improve disease activity.
- Chronic heart failure: improvements in exercise capacity and symptoms yet not enough data available.
- Common cold: not enough data available.
- Fibromyalgia: may improve pain and sleep yet not enough data available.
- Juvenile idiopathic arthritis: pain reductions reported yet not enough data available.

- Labour: reductions in pain and anxiety yet not enough data available.
- Neck pain: not enough data available.
- Neuromotor impairment, children: some positive reports exist yet data are not convincing.
- Osteoarthritis: some positive findings yet not enough data available.
- Pressure ulcers: not enough data available.

😕 *Unlikely to be beneficial*
- Psoriasis vulgaris: saline water is unlikely to have any beneficial effects.

Risks
- *Contraindications:* acute heart failure, decompensated heart failure, acute skin conditions, severe varicose veins.
- *Precautions/warnings:* none known.
- *Adverse effects:* applications with water that is too hot or too cold may cause burns or hypothermia. May cause exacerbation of chronic venous insufficiency.

Conclusions

- There is some evidence of effectiveness for chronic venous insufficiency, chronic low back pain, and rheumatoid arthritis
- Adverse events are on record but these are usually infrequent and of mild nature if contraindications are observed
- The risk–benefit balance is likely to be positive for spa/balneotherapy in chronic low back pain and rheumatoid arthritis, and for hydrotherapeutic interventions in chronic venous insufficiency

Table 3.5 Systematic up-to-date review where hydrotherapy has been found likely to be beneficial

Condition	Source	No. of trials/ patients	Original conclusion
Low back pain	Rheumatology 2006; **45**:880–4	N=5/n=580	Even though the data are scarce, there is encouraging evidence suggesting that spa therapy and balneotherapy may be effective for treating patients with low back pain

Further reading

Lange U, Muller-Ladner U, Schmidt KL. Balneotherapy in rheumatic diseases—an overview of novel and known aspects. *Rheumatol Int* 2006; **26**:497–9.
Reid Campion M. *Hydrotherapy Principles and Practice*. Oxford: Butterworth Heinemann, 1997.

Hypnotherapy

Definition
The induction of a trance-like state to facilitate relaxation and make use of enhanced suggestibility to treat psychological and medical conditions and affect behavioural changes.

The concept
The first therapeutic use of hypnotic practices has been attributed to the Austrian physician Franz Anton Mesmer in 1778. Hypnotherapy aims at gaining self-control over behaviour, emotions, or physiological processes. This is achieved by induction of the hypnotic trance where the patient's focus of attention is directed inwards, thereby allowing easier access to the non-critical unconscious mind which is more receptive to suggestion. Hypnosis is usually associated with a deep state of relaxation. The means by which hypnotic suggestion enables involuntary processes such as skin temperature, heart rate and gut secretions to be deliberately controlled is not fully understood.

Related techniques
Self-hypnosis, imagery, autogenic training, meditation, relaxation.

Treatment
Sessions typically last between 30 and 90 minutes. The initial visit involves the gathering of history and discussion about hypnosis, suggestion, and the client's expectations of the therapy. Tests for hypnotic suggestibility may also be conducted. Hypnotic induction may or may not be part of the first session. The hypnotic state is achieved by first relaxing the body, then shifting attention away from the external environment towards a narrow range of objects or ideas suggested by the therapist. Sometimes hypnotherapy is carried out in group settings, e.g. antenatal classes as preparation for labour. An average course is 6–12 weekly sessions.

Clinical bottom line
Benefits

☺ *Beneficial*
- Labour: beneficial for pain relief.

☺ *Likely to be beneficial*
- Anxiety: seems to improve procedure-related anxiety in children and adults, distress in paediatric oncology patients.
- Headache: although data not uniformly positive the majority of trials suggest benefits.
- Insomnia: trials methodologically limited but overall suggest effectiveness.
- Irritable bowel syndrome: seems to improve symptoms and quality of life.
- Nausea/vomiting, chemotherapy-induced: helpful for anticipatory and chemotherapy-induced nausea in children and adolescents.
- Pain management: seems to improve postoperative pain, chronic pain, procedure-related pain.

🙁 *Unknown effectiveness*
- Asthma, symptoms and lung function: not enough data available.
- Cancer, palliation: may relief pain, nausea/vomiting, fatigue yet more data required.
- Conversion disorder: more data required.
- Depression: may improve symptoms yet not enough data available.
- Eczema: severity but not enough data available.
- Erectile dysfunction: improvements in sexual function but not enough data available.
- Fibromyalgia: may have analgesic effects yet more data are required.
- Hair loss: encouraging but only preliminary data available.
- Herpes labialis: may reduce intensity.
- Hypertension: may reduce blood pressure in the short term yet not enough data available.
- Nausea/vomiting, postoperative: women undergoing breast surgery but not enough data available.
- Nausea/vomiting, pregnancy-related: not enough data available.
- Non-ulcer dyspepsia: not enough data available.
- Overweight/obesity: as adjunct to cognitive–behavioural therapy small body weight reduction.
- Post-traumatic conditions: not enough data available.
- Psoriasis: not enough data available.
- Rheumatoid arthritis: pain management but not enough data available.
- Seasonal allergic rhinitis: not enough data available.
- Schizophrenia: data scarce and methodologically limited.
- Stroke: evidence is not convincing for stroke rehabilitation.
- Tinnitus: subjective symptoms but not enough data available.
- Vaginismus: not enough data available.
- Wound/fracture healing: not enough data available.

Likely to be ineffective
- Alcohol dependence: likely to be ineffective.
- Epilepsy: likely to be ineffective.
- Smoking cessation: likely to be ineffective.

Risks
- *Contraindications:* psychosis, personality disorders.
- *Precautions/warnings:* information elicited under hypnosis is subject to confabulation, epilepsy, very young children.
- *Adverse effects:* recovering repressed memories can be painful and psychological problems may be exacerbated. False memory syndrome has been reported. Studies investigating negative consequences of hypnosis have concluded that when practised by a clinically trained professional, it is safe.

Conclusions

- Hypnotherapy has analgesic effects and appears to reduce pain-associated anxiety. There is also evidence that it is helpful for patients with irritable bowel syndrome, insomnia, and nausea
- The possibility of adverse effects has to be considered but it seems safe
- The risk–benefit balance for hypnotherapy in the management of a range of pain syndromes is positive or likely to be positive: it is also likely to be positive for irritable bowel syndrome, chemotherapy-induced nausea and anxiety

Table 3.6 Systematic up-to-date reviews where hypnotherapy has been found to be beneficial or likely to be beneficial

Condition	Source	No. of trials/ patients	Original conclusion
Anxiety	J Pain Symptom Manage 2006; **1**: 70-84	N=7/n=293	… hypnosis has potential as a clinically valuable intervention that could contribute to the management of procedure-related pain and distress in pediatric cancer patients
Irritable bowel syndrome	Aliment Pharmacol Ther 2006; **24**: 769-80	N=6/n=223	The published evidence suggests that hypnotherapy is effective in the management of IBS
Labour, pain management	Cochrane Database Syst Rev 2006; **4**: CD003521	N=5/n=729	… hypnosis may be beneficial for the management of pain during labour: however, the number of women studied has been small
Pain management	Cochrane Database Syst Rev 2006; **4**: CD005179	N=5/n=216	Overall, there is sufficient evidence to support the efficacy of distraction, hypnosis, and combined CBT in reducing pain and distress in children and adolescents undergoing needle procedures

Further reading

Anbar RD. Hypnosis: an important multifaceted therapy. J Pediatr 2006; **149**:438–9.
James U. Clinical Hypnosis Textbook: A Guide for Practical Intervention. Oxford: Radcliffe Publishing, 2005.
The British Association of Medical Hypnosis. http://www.bamh.org.uk/

Imagery

Definition

A mind–body technique that involves using the imagination and mental images to encourage physical healing, promote relaxation, and bring about a change in attitude or behaviour.

Concept

A visualization technique that is based on the notion that the mind can affect the body. Stimulating the brain through visualization may have direct effects on endocrine and nervous systems and may lead to changes in immune and other functions.

Related techniques

Meditation, hypnosis.

Treatment

Imagery is usually taught in small classes. Sessions begin with general relaxation exercises and then move on to more specific visualization techniques. Patients will be led to build detailed images and if a specific medical condition exists, may be asked to picture the body free of that condition. Athletes or performers may picture themselves moving well and competing or performing perfectly. Sessions last generally 20–30 minutes, once or twice weekly for several weeks.

Clinical bottom line

Benefit

😃 *Likely to be beneficial*

- Cancer: seems to be psycho-supportive, decrease anxiety and depression, and increase comfort.
- Fibromyalgia: seems to reduce current pain and anxiety.
- Postoperative pain: seems to reduce pain and analgesic requirements.

😐 *Unknown effectiveness*

- AIDS/HIV infection: not enough data available.
- Abdominal pain: combined with progressive muscle relaxation may decrease the number of days with pain in children.
- Asthma: may improve symptoms yet data contradictory.
- Bulimia nervosa: may reduce bingeing and purging yet not enough data available.
- Burns: reduction in the self-reporting of pain yet not enough data available.
- Burns: may reduce the self-reporting of pain in children during debridement.
- Cancer: may relieve pain but data contradictory.
- Cardiovascular disease: in combination with prayer, music therapy and touch therapy may lower 6-month mortality.
- Chronic low back pain: not enough data available.
- Chronic obstructive pulmonary disease: may increase oxygen saturation but not enough data available.

- Depression: encouraging preliminary evidence but not enough data available.
- End of life: relaxation/imagery can improve pain from oral mucositis but not enough data available.
- Headache: might improve symptoms when used as an adjunct therapy but not enough data available.
- Multiple sclerosis: not enough data available.
- Neuropathic pain: may reduce phantom limb pain and improve function but not enough data available.
- Osteoarthritis: may improve quality of life but not enough data available.
- Posttraumatic stress disorder: may improve sleep quality, decrease chronic nightmares and stress symptoms but not enough data available.
- Sleep: may improve sleep quality in critically ill patients but not enough data available.
- Stroke: may promote the relearning of daily tasks but not enough data available.
- Sympathetic dystrophy: not enough data available.

🙁 *Unlikely to be beneficial*
- Nausea/vomiting, chemotherapy-induced.

💀 *Likely to be ineffective or harmful*
- End-stage renal disease: unlikely to be effective.
- Intravenous insertion pain: unlikely to reduce pain.
- Labour pain: unlikely to reduce pain.

Risks
- *Contraindications:* severe mental illness. Latent psychosis and personality disorders, as these may become overt with introspection.
- *Precautions/warnings:* should only be used as an adjunct to standard therapy.
- *Adverse effects:* none.

Conclusions

- Data suggests that imagery is likely to be beneficial for cancer, fibromyalgia, and postoperative pain
- Imagery is almost risk-free
- The risk–benefit balance for the above conditions is likely to be positive

Further reading
Hall E, Hall C, Stradling P, Young D. *Guided Imagery: Creative Interventions in Counselling and Psychotherapy.* Thousand Oaks, CA: Sage Publications, 2006.

Massage

Definition

A method of manipulating the soft tissue of whole body areas (primary focus on 'Swedish massage'). Considered a complementary therapy in many countries, yet in some European countries (e.g. Germany) massage continues to be part of conventional medicine.

The concept

Massage is applied using various manual techniques, applying pressure and traction. The friction of the hands and the mechanical pressure exerted on cutaneous and subcutaneous structures affect the body. The circulation of blood and lymph is generally enhanced, resulting in increased oxygen supply. Direct mechanical pressure and effects mediated by the nervous system beneficially affect areas of increased muscular tension.

Related techniques

Aromatherapy, reflexology, shiatsu.

Treatment

The patient's medical history will be assessed to get an overall impression of the medical status and possible contraindications. Patients are normally treated unclothed with a sheet or towel provided. Usually the massage is performed on a specially designed massage couch. Therapists often use oil to facilitate movement of their hands over the patient's body. The duration of individual treatment sessions varies, but will typically be about 30 minutes. Sometimes sessions are followed by other treatments such as hot packs, which essentially applies external heat. Usually 1–2 sessions weekly for a treatment period of 4–8 weeks.

Clinical bottom line

:☺: *Beneficial*
- Anxiety: improves anxiety of various causes.

☺ *Likely to be beneficial*
- AIDS/HIV infection: may improve quality of life.
- Back pain: seems to improve symptoms in subacute and chronic non-specific low back pain.
- Constipation: abdominal massage could be a promising option.
- Depression, adults: seems to improve symptoms.
- Labour: may improve pain and anxiety.
- Musculoskeletal pain: vibratory massage seems of benefit.
- Shoulder pain: data for pain relief are encouraging.

☹ *Unknown effectiveness*
- Alzheimer's disease: not enough data available.
- Attention deficit hyperactivity disorder: not enough data available.
- Asthma: not enough data available.

- Cancer, breast: may improve immune function and nausea due to chemotherapy but not enough data available.
- Cancer: data are for pain relief contradictory, for fatigue not enough data available.
- Cardiovascular disease: may improve wellbeing.
- Cystic fibrosis: may be useful as an adjunct treatment but data scarce.
- Dementia: may improve symptoms yet not enough data available.
- Depression, children and adolescents: not enough data available.
- Diarrhoea: not enough data available.
- Fibromyalgia: may improve pain, depression, and quality of life but not enough data available.
- Headache, tension-type: not enough data available.
- Insomnia: may improve sleep quality but not enough data available.
- Irritable bowel syndrome: not enough data available.
- Migraine: may improve frequency and sleep quality, not enough data available.
- Multiple sclerosis: preliminary data suggest improvements of anxiety and depression but not enough data available.
- Nausea/vomiting, chemotherapy-induced: data are conflicting.
- Neck disorders, mechanical: data are inconsistent.
- Osteoarthritis: may improve pain stiffness and function but not enough data available.
- Post-exercise muscle soreness: does not affect duration of pain, loss of strength and function yet not enough data available.
- Premenstrual syndrome: not enough data available.
- Smoking cessation: not enough data available.
- Stroke: may reduce pain and anxiety but not enough data available.
- Tendinitis: not enough data available.
- Upper extremity work-related disorders: data few and methodologically limited.

🗙 *Likely to be ineffective or harmful*
- Eczema: no evidence of effectiveness.
- Preterm and/or low birth-weight infants: likely to be ineffective for promoting growth and development.
- Healthy infants: likely to be ineffective for promoting growth in infants under age 6 months.

Risks
- *Contraindications:* phlebitis, deep vein thrombosis, burns, skin infections, eczema, open wounds, bone fractures, advanced osteoporosis.
- *Precautions/warnings:* cancer, myocardial infarction, osteoporosis, pregnancy.
- *Adverse effects:* rare: bone fractures, organ liver rupture.
- *Interactions:* possible with oils used for massage.

Conclusions

- Data indicate that massage is beneficial in anxiety as well as likely to be beneficial in conditions such as AIDS/HIV, constipation, depression, labour pain, back pain and musculoskeletal pain
- Few risks are involved
- The risk–benefit balance is positive for the above indications. Its relaxing effects may have some albeit non-specific influence on the wellbeing of most patients

Further reading

Jewell Rich G. *Massage Therapy: The Evidence for Practice*. St Louis: Mosby, 2002.
The General Council for Massage Therapy. http://www.gcmt.org.uk/

Meditation

Definition
A conscious mental process aimed at focusing the attention and bringing about a state of self-awareness and inner calm. It comprises a very diverse array of techniques (e.g. transcendental meditation, TM; Sahaja yoga/meditation, mindfulness meditation, MM; meditative prayer) which are based on listening to breath, repeating a mantra, detaching from the thought process or self-directed mental practices. Most forms of meditation originated within the major religions particularly those of the East. In the West it became popular during the 1960s and 1970s when it became associated with hippy and pop culture. It continues to be taught in religious, cultic and non-cultic contexts: the latter includes forms developed for therapeutic purposes.

Concept
Meditation is aimed at inducing physiological changes, i.e. the relaxation response. Numerous studies report changes in physiological parameters such as oxygen consumption, respiration rate, heart rate and brain activity during meditation. Although these changes may have positive health effects, specific mechanisms remain unknown.

Related techniques
Benson's relaxation response (BRR), qigong, yoga.

Treatment
Meditation is mainly taught by religious or quasi-religious groups. TM is promoted by a worldwide organization, while MM was developed within a healthcare context. Following initial instruction carried out over several sessions, meditators are expected to practise regularly twice daily for 15–20 minutes. The prophylactic and therapeutic effects are expected to accrue from continued daily practice.

Clinical bottom line
Benefits

☺ *Likely to be beneficial*
- Anxiety: TM, positive effects on trait anxiety.
- Stress: passage meditation and MM may reduce symptoms.

☻ *Unknown effectiveness*
- Asthma: Sahaja meditation, not enough data available.
- Chronic heart failure: improvement in quality of life but not enough data available.
- Cognitive function: TM, studies have severe methodological limitations.
- Constipation: more data required.
- Epilepsy: data are scarce and have methodological weaknesses.
- Fibromyalgia, depressive symptoms: MM, not enough data available.
- Hypertension: TM, data are contradictory and methodologically limited.
- Irritable bowel syndrome: only few data available which also require independent replication.

- Menopausal symptoms: BRR, encouraging results but not enough data available.
- Premenstrual syndrome: data encouraging but not sufficient.
- Psoriasis: MM, not enough data available.

Risks

- *Contraindications:* could theoretically create conditions in the brain conducive to epilepsy.
- *Precautions/warnings:* people with pre-existing mental health problems should be closely supervised.
- *Adverse effects:* uncomfortable kinesthetic sensations, mild dissociation and psychosis-like symptoms, exacerbation of pre-existing psychiatric illnesses.
- *Interactions:* none known.

Conclusions

- Meditation is likely to be effective in improving anxiety and reducing stress symptoms
- No serious risks have been reported but patients with mental health problems should be monitored
- The risk–benefit balance for stress and anxiety is likely to be positive

Further reading

Canter PH. The therapeutic effects of meditation. *BMJ* 2003; **326**:1049–50.

Music therapy

Definition

The use of music by an accredited professional to achieve individualized therapeutic goals. The most basic distinction is between receptive (listening to music played by the therapist or recorded music) and active music (patients are involved in the music-making).

Concept

Sensations that accompany music therapy may activate limbic or other areas of the brain related to the reward and motivation circuitry (limbic-cortical circuits). Secondary physiological changes and bodily reactions may follow, i.e., autoregulatory mind/body reactions such as an influence on hemispheric dominance, changes in autonomic nervous system activity, relaxation effects on vital functions such as breath, respiratory rate, blood pressure, and cardiac output. Analgesic and anxiolytic properties of music are mainly due to the lowering of stress levels and stress hormone production similar to the relaxation response. There are wide variations in individual music preferences which have a strong impact on the physiological effects of music.

Treatment

Since music therapists serve a wide variety of persons with many different types of complaints there is no overall typical session. In pain management, for example, mainly receptive music therapy is used while active music therapy is most common in mental health. The duration of receptive music therapy for pain can be between a single session, for example before, during or after surgery, to a series of sessions over several weeks for chronic pain patients. Active music therapy is used as a form of expression in, for example, mental health or palliative care.

Clinical bottom line

Benefits

:☺: *Beneficial*

- Anxiety, perioperative and procedural: useful adjunct in reducing anxiety and sedative requirements, decreasing blood pressure, improving physiological parameters.
- Psychopathology: best results for behavioural and developmental disorders.
- Stress: reduces anxiety and enhances relaxation response.

☺ *Likely to be beneficial*

- Mood: might improve mood in a range of conditions.
- Pain, perioperative and procedural: encouraging results for music therapy as an adjunct therapy.
- Schizophrenia: in addition to standard care, improves global state.

☹ *Unknown effectiveness*

- Anaerobic performance: data are contradictory.
- Anxiety and stress, after acute myocardial infarction: data contradictory.

- Autism spectrum disorder: auditory integration therapy, data contradictory.
- Back pain: not enough data available.
- Cancer: clinical music therapy might improve quality of life but not enough data available.
- Cystic fibrosis: recorded music as an adjunct during routine chest physiotherapy, not enough data available.
- Dementia: studies are methodologically too limited to draw any useful conclusions.
- Depression: encouraging results but data scarce.
- Epilepsy: may reduce seizure frequency yet not enough data available.
- Fibromyalgia: not enough data available.
- Insomnia: not enough data available.
- Multiple sclerosis: strengthening of respiratory muscles through coordination of breath and speech but not enough data available.
- Nausea and vomiting, chemotherapy-induced: not enough data available.
- Osteoarthritis: not enough data available.
- Parkinson's disease: additional active music therapy might improve motor, affective, and behavioural functions but not enough data available.
- Premature infants: live music therapy might improve heart rate and sleep but not enough data available.
- Stroke: additional active music therapy supports neurorehabilitation of motor skills.

🙁 *Unlikely to be beneficial*
- Labour: no effects on pain reported.

🗙 *Likely to be ineffective or harmful*
- Nausea/vomiting, postoperative: no beneficial effects.

Risks
- *Contraindications:* none known.
- *Precautions/warnings:* none known.
- *Adverse effects:* none known.
- *Interactions:* none known.

Conclusions

- Music therapy as an adjunct therapy has positive effects on anxiety and stress as well as psychopathological disorders; it might improve pain symptoms, schizophrenia, and mood in a range of conditions
- No risks have been reported
- The risk–benefit balance for the above conditions is positive or likely to be positive

Table 3.7 Systematic up-to-date reviews where music therapy has been found to be beneficial or likely to be beneficial

Condition	Source	No. of trials/ patients	Original conclusion
Psychopathology	*J Child Psychol Psychiatry* 2004; **45**:1054–63	N=11/n=188	Music therapy has a medium-to-large positive effect on clinically relevant outcomes ... Effects tended to be greater for behavioural and developmental disorders than for emotional disorders
Schizophrenia	*Cochrane Database Syst Rev* 2005; **2**: CD004025	N=4/n=266	Music therapy as an addition to standard care helps people with schizophrenia to improve their global state and may also improve mental state and functioning

Further reading

Bunt L. Clinical and Therapeutic Uses of Music. In Hargreaves DJ, North AC, eds. *The Social Psychology of Music.* New York: Oxford University Press, 1997.
The British Society for Music Therapy. http://www.bsmt.org/

Naturopathy

Definition

An eclectic system of healthcare, which integrates elements of complementary and conventional medicine to support and enhance self-healing processes.

Concept

Naturopathy is based on the belief that health is influenced by nature's own healing power, which is understood as an inherent property of the living organism. Ill health is viewed as a direct consequence of violating general principles of a healthy lifestyle. These principles, including a diet that is rich in fresh fruit and vegetables and a sufficient amount of physical exercise, are well recognized in conventional medicine. The different therapeutic interventions and techniques include herbal medicine, and iridology (as a diagnostic technique) as well as physical treatments (e.g. hydrotherapy, spinal manipulation) and others. The scientific rationale varies according to each individual modality. For some (e.g. iridology) a plausible scientific rationale is lacking, while for others (e.g. physical exercise) the rationale is supported by science.

Related techniques

Hydrotherapy, physical medicine, physiotherapy.

Treatment

During an initial consultation the naturopath will usually take a detailed medical history of the patient. This will also include questions relating to lifestyle and diet and may be followed by a more conventional diagnostic evaluation, including laboratory analyses. According to the diagnosed condition, the treatment plan will vary but often includes a change in lifestyle. The treatment of a particular condition may vary between practitioners. Follow-up appointments are arranged as necessary and medicines and regimen reviewed and changed if appropriate. Depending largely on the nature and severity of the condition treatment consists generally of 1–2 appointments per week for a treatment period of one to several weeks.

Clinical bottom line

The clinical evidence has to be evaluated according to each individual therapy (📖 see respective chapters). There is clinical evidence from randomized clinical trials and systematic reviews for some elements of naturopathy, such as certain herbal extracts. For other elements there is evidence against their use such as iridology. The effectiveness of the totality of the naturopathic approach has not been evaluated in randomized clinical trials.

Risks

- *Contraindications:* contraindications and precautions vary for each individual therapy (📖 see respective chapters) and often include pregnancy and lactation.

- *Precautions/warnings:* precautions may vary for each individual therapy (📖 see respective chapters).
- *Adverse effects:* the risk of adverse effects exists. The reader is referred to the respective chapters in this book and the conventional medical literature.
- *Interactions:* possible interactions, for instance between different herbal preparations or with conventional drugs or other intervention, should be considered (📖 see respective chapters) and relevant patients should be closely monitored. Patients should be asked about self-prescription drug use.

Conclusions

- The benefit has to be assessed for each treatment individually (📖 see respective chapters)
- The possibility of adverse effects exists
- The risk–benefit ratio has to be assessed for each treatment individually (📖 see respective chapters)

Further reading

Jagtenberg T, Evans S, Grant A, Howden I, Lewis M, Singer J. Evidence-based medicine and naturopathy. *J Altern Complement Med* 2006; **12**:323–8.
The British Naturopathic Association. http://www.naturopaths.org.uk/

Neural therapy

Definition
A treatment originating from Germany which involves injections (often subcutaneous) of local anaesthetics (e.g. Novocain®) into specific areas called 'irritation zones' (often old scars).

Concept
Neural therapy aims to deblock reflex pathways and stimulate auto-regulatory mechanisms. Proponents believe that every chronic condition can be caused by 'irritation zones' which can be created by every disease or injury and that injections can eliminate these 'irritation zones'.

Related techniques
Acupuncture, local anaesthesia, trigger point injections.

Treatment
Typically a conventional medical history is taken followed by a physical examination. In particular, 'irritation zones' (e.g. old scars) are searched for. The results determine the treatment which usually would consist of injections with local anaesthetics, often under the skin but sometimes also into deeper structures (e.g. around internal organs). Therapists sometimes observe that this cures a problem within seconds ('*Sekunden-Phänomen*'). If not, a series of treatment may consist of 6–12 sessions.

Clinical bottom line
Benefits
😑 *Unknown effectiveness*
- Back pain: not enough data available.
- Multiple sclerosis: preliminary data show a reduction of subjective symptoms but not enough data available.

Risks
- *Contraindications:* allergic reactions to local anaesthetic.
- *Precautions/warnings:* needle phobia.
- *Adverse effects:* allergic reactions, puncture of internal organs.
- *Interactions:* depends on local anaesthetic employed.

Conclusions
- Effectiveness has not been adequately demonstrated for any condition
- Only minor risks have been reported
- Risk–benefit balance fails to be positive

Further reading
Kidd RF. *Neural Therapy: Applied Neurophysiology and Other Topics.* Ontario, Canada: RF Kidd Books, 2005.

Osteopathy

Definition
Manual therapy involving manipulation of soft tissue and mobilization/manipulation of joints.

Concept
Adequate alignment of the musculoskeletal system is viewed as crucial for blood and lymph flow, as well as organ function. Osteopaths restore malalignment through various manual techniques, particularly mobilization.

Related techniques
Chiropractic, manual therapy, spinal manipulation/mobilization, massage, craniosacral therapy.

Treatment
Osteopaths take a medical history and conduct a thorough physical examination, particularly of the spine. This is followed by manual treatments, which are typically less forceful than those of chiropractors (manipulation). One session may last about 30 minutes. A full course may consist of around 6 sessions; more for chronic conditions.

Clinical bottom line
Benefits
Likely to be effective
- Back pain: particularly acute/subacute.
- Shoulder pain: might speed up recovery but studies are not uniformly positive.

😐 *Unknown effectiveness*
- Fibromyalgia: not enough data available.
- Menopause: hot flushes, not enough data available.
- Pneumonia: not enough data available.
- Post-operative pain: enhanced effect of morphine, not enough data.
- Postural asymmetry of infants: not enough data available.
- Rehabilitation after knee or hip arthroplasty: not enough data available.
- Tennis elbow: pain intensity, function, not enough data available.

☠ *Likely to be ineffective or harmful*
- Primary or secondary dysmenorrhoea: likely to be ineffective.

Risks
- *Contraindications:* osteoporosis, neoplasms and infections of the bone, bleeding abnormalities.
- *Precautions/warnings:* none known.
- *Adverse effects:* vertebral artery dissection (after high-velocity thrusts to the upper spine).
- *Interactions:* none known.

Conclusions

- Likely to be effective for treatment of mechanical acute/subacute back pain and shoulder pain
- Reasonably good safety record
- Risk–benefit balance is likely to be positive for treating acute/subacute back pain and shoulder pain

Table 3.8 Systematic up-to-date reviews where osteopathy has been found likely to be beneficial

Condition	Source	No. of trials/ patients	Original conclusion
Back pain	*BMC Musculoskelet Disord* 2005; **6**:43	N=6/n=525	Osteopathic manipulative treatment reduces back pain ... [more] than expected from placebo

Further reading

Lederman E. *The Science and Practice of Manual Therapy*. Edinburgh: Churchill Livingstone, 2005.
The General Osteopathic Council. http://www.osteopathy.org.uk/

Qigong

Definition
An Asian healing art that uses gentle, focused exercises for mind and body to increase and restore the flow of qi (life energy) or accumulate qi with the aim of encouraging and accelerating the healing process.

Concept
Qigong (pronounced /chee-gong/) consists of two main types of practice, internal and external, and aims to restore health through removing blockages of qi. Internal qigong is self-directed and involves the use of movements and meditation. It can be performed with or without the presence of a teacher. External qigong is performed by a trained practitioner using the hands and any part of body to direct qi energy onto the patient. Two main aspects are involved in qigong practice, controlled breathing with slow body movements as an aerobic exercise and relaxation. The exercises are physical stimuli with effects on the cardiovascular and muscular system and may enhance function, balance and coordination.

Related techniques
Tai chi, Danjun (Tantien) breathing, Zen meditation, Reiki, therapeutic touch, Johrei, spiritual healing.

Treatment
Qigong is taught on an individual basis or in groups. Qigong is a lifelong endeavour and regular practice is essential in achieving beneficial effects. Treatment may differ in duration but usually takes 30 minutes. Daily practice is ideal and at least twice weekly sessions are recommended. Usually, external qigong is for the beginner who cannot yet perform internal qigong, which is thought to be superior.

Clinical bottom line
Benefits

😊 *Likely to be beneficial*
- Hypertension: systolic blood pressure.

😐 *Unknown effectiveness*
- Cancer: pain reduction yet not enough data available.
- Depression: may improve mood, self-efficacy, and personal well being but not enough data available.
- Diabetes, type 2: insulin resistance yet not enough data available.
- Drug dependence: might reduce withdrawal symptoms of heroin addicts but not enough data available.
- Fibromyalgia: in addition to mindfulness meditation pain reduction yet not enough data available.
- Late-stage complex regional pain syndrome: not enough data available.
- Migraine, tension-type headache: not enough data available.
- Parkinson's disease: improvement of motor symptoms yet not enough data available.
- Pre-menstrual syndrome: reduction in pain yet data methodologically limited.

on therapy

eliciting the 'relaxation response' of the autonomic nervous

ation therapy such as progressive muscle relaxation are
citing the relaxation response, resulting in decreases in
nption, heart rate, respiration, and skeletal muscle activity
malizing of blood supply to the muscles. Other relaxation
olve passive muscle relaxation, refocusing, breathing con-
y. With imagery-based relaxation, the idea is to visualize
ace or situation associated with relaxation and comfort.
ues have also been reported to be effective in diffusing

niques

ning, biofeedback, hypnotherapy, meditation. Many CAM
nclude an element of relaxation.

ive muscle relaxation, subjects usually lie on their back with
le in a quiet environment. Occasionally a sitting posture in a
hair is adopted instead. Muscle groups are systematically
en relaxed in a predetermined order. In the early stages, an
will be devoted to a single muscle group. With practice it
ble to combine muscle groups and then eventually relax
ll at once. With progressive muscle relaxation, several
y practice is needed in order to be able to evoke the relaxa-
within seconds.

om line

sensitization for agoraphobia and panic disorder, anxiety
vith cancer and in patients undergoing medical interven-
s radiation therapy.
provement through progressive muscle relaxation training,
-based stress reduction, and relaxation tapes.
iting, chemotherapy-induced: preventing nausea and
ore, during, and after chemotherapy.

* beneficial
iation: seems to reduce anxiety, depression, and vasomotor
articularly in breast cancer patients.
similar effects as cognitive behaviour therapy.
esults are contradictory but most rigorous studies suggest
fect on pain.
on: small effects for systolic and diastolic blood pressure.

- Rehabilitation, coronary artery disease: improvement in physical performance and activity yet not enough data available.
- Shoulder-arm pain: not enough data available.

😟 *Unlikely to be beneficial*
- Overweight/obesity: unlikely to reduce body weight.

Risks
- *Contraindications:* largely based on common sense (e.g. severe osteoporosis, severe heart conditions, acute back pain, knee problems, sprains and fractures). Usually it can be practised during pregnancy and lactation.
- *Precautions/warnings:* before starting qigong older individuals should be carefully examined for any of the above or other contraindications.
- *Adverse effects:* rare, but may include delayed-onset muscle soreness. When practised inappropriately, it may induce abnormal psychosomatic responses and mental disorders.

Conclusions

- There is evidence that qigong might be effective in patients with hypertension
- No serious adverse events are on record
- The risk–benefit balance is likely to be positive for hypertension

Table 3.9 Systematic up-to-date review where qigong has been found to be likely to be beneficial

Condition	Source	No. of trials/patients	Original conclusion
Hypertension	*J Hypertension* 2007; **25**:1525–32	N=12/n=1218	There is some encouraging evidence to suggest that qigong is effective for lowering systolic blood pressure

Further reading

Johnson JA. *Chinese Medical Qigong Therapy: A Comprehensive Clinical Guide.* California: International Institute of Medical Qigong, 2000.

Reflexology

Definition
Treatment employing manual pressure to specific areas of the body, usually the feet, which are thought to correspond to internal organs with a view to generate positive health effects.

Concept
The sole of the foot is believed to be a map where the entire body is represented. Reflexologists palpate the foot looking for signs of tenderness or grittiness, which would indicate weaknesses in the corresponding organs. Massaging these areas is claimed to influence specific organ function, reduce stress, eliminate toxins, rebalance the body's energy, improve circulation, or promote metabolic homeostasis.

Related techniques
Acupressure, shiatsu, Korean hand massage.

Treatment
The therapist takes a medical history, palpates the foot and subsequently applies manual pressure and massage. Each session lasts 45–60 minutes. Typically treatments are weekly. A full course may include 6–8 sessions.

Clinical bottom line
Benefits
😊 *Unknown effectiveness*
- Anxiety: short-term symptom reduction, not enough data available.
- Chronic obstructive pulmonary disease: symptom control, not enough data.
- Dementia, agitation: not enough data available.
- Depression, symptom control: not enough data available.
- Detrusor overactivity, diurnal micturation: not enough data available.
- Diabetes, glucose control: not enough data available.
- Headache, pain intensity: encouraging but few and methodologically limited data available.
- Multiple sclerosis, motor sensory and urinary symptoms: not enough data available.
- Insomnia: not enough data available.
- Leg oedema during pregnancy: not enough data available.
- Premenstrual syndrome, symptom control: not enough data available.
- Smoking cessation: might improve withdrawal symptoms but not enough data available.

😣 *Unlikely to be beneficial*
- Asthma, attack frequency.
- Cancer palliation, quality of life.
- Irritable bowel syndrome: seems ineffective for improving pain, distension and constipation/diarrhoea.
- Labour: no effects on onset or duration of labour.

☠ *Likely to be ineffective or harmful*
- Constipation: frequency of bowel

Risks
- *Contraindications:* gout, leg ulcers,
- *Precautions/warnings:* some reflex inadequate competence.
- *Adverse effects:* fatigue, changes in
- *Interactions:* interference with insu

Conclusions
- The effectiveness of reflexology
- Good safety record
- Risk–benefit balance fails to be p

Further reading
Mackareth P, Tiran D (Eds). *Clinical Reflexology: A* Livingstone, 2002.

Relaxat

Definition
Techniques f system.

Concept
Forms of re effective in oxygen cons and in the r techniques trol, or ima oneself in a These tech muscle tens

Related te
Autogenic interventio

Treatme
With prog arms to the comfortabl contracted entire sess becomes p entire boc months of tion respo

Clinical
Benefits
😊 *Bene*
- Anxiety associa tions su
- Insomn mindfu
- Nause vomiti

😊 *Likely*
- Cance sympt
- Depre
- Heada a posi
- Hyper

- Ischaemic heart disease: seems to improve outcomes indicative of enhanced recovery.
- Low back pain, chronic: short-term pain relief and functional improvement.
- Menopause: seems to reduce the frequency of hot flush symptoms but evidence is inconsistent regarding the best type of relaxation method.
- Migraine: it seems to benefit adults when used in combination with biofeedback or alone.
- Rheumatoid arthritis: may be beneficial in pain management.

😕 *Unknown effectiveness*
- Asthma, adults: may reduce medication needs but studies methodologically limitated.
- Asthma, children: may improve pulmonary function but studies small and methodologically limited.
- Chronic fatigue syndrome: inferior to cognitive-behavioural therapy.
- Chronic heart failure: improvement in quality of life but not enough data available.
- Chronic obstructive pulmonary disease, dyspnoea: not enough data available.
- Crohn's disease: may reduce healthcare utilization but not enough data available.
- Coronary syndrome X: encouraging data but not enough data available.
- Fatigue, cancer related: not enough data available.
- Neck pain: might improve pain more than usual care but not enough data available.
- Night eating syndrome: encouraging data but not enough data available.
- Pain, acute, chronic: data are conflicting.
- Phobia, social: combined with cognitive therapy may lead to improvement.
- Premenstrual syndrome: not enough data available.
- Preterm labour outcome: encouraging data but not enough data available.
- Smoking cessation: may reduce stress during nicotine withdrawal but not enough data available.
- Temporomandibular disorder: may improve symptoms but data limited.
- Ulcerative colitis: data are encouraging but not convincing for progressive muscle relaxation.

🔀 *Likely to be ineffective or harmful*
- Cancer, treatment: likely to be ineffective as 'breast cancer cure'.
- Drug dependency: not effective for withdrawal symptoms.
- Epilepsy: no effect on seizure frequency.
- Irritable bowel syndrome: likely to be ineffective.
- Non-ulcer dyspepsia: likely to be ineffective.

Risks
- *Contraindications:* schizophrenic or actively psychotic patients.
- *Precautions/warnings:* techniques requiring inward focusing may intensify depressed mood.
- *Adverse effects:* none known.

Conclusions

- Relaxation techniques may be useful for treating anxiety disorders and conditions with a psychosomatic element although these may not be long-term. They are likely to be beneficial for a range of conditions
- Relaxation therapies are almost risk-free
- The risk–benefit balance for the above conditions is positive or likely to be positive

Further reading

Kwekkeboom KL, Gretarsdottir E. Systematic review of relaxation interventions for pain. *J Nurs Scholarsh* 2006; **38**:269–77.

Payne R. *Relaxation Techniques: A Practical Handbook for the Health Care Professional.* Edinburgh: Churchill Livingstone, 2004.

Shiatsu

Definition
Therapy of Japanese origin, in which pressure is applied usually with the fingers or hands to certain points of the body. In Japanese, the term shiatsu literally means finger (*shi*) pressure (*atsu*).

Concept
Shiatsu involves finger, palm or elbow pressure, stretching, massaging and other manual techniques. A disease state is believed to occur when the energy flow is blocked, deficient, or in excess. A goal of shiatsu is to restore the normal flow of life energy using various manual techniques. The soft tissue manipulation of cutaneous and subcutaneous structures may improve blood circulation and may reduce muscle pain and tension. Shiatsu could thus be a method of affecting the nervous and muscular systems, similar to massage and acupuncture.

Related techniques
Bodywork therapy, massage.

Treatment
Shiatsu is practised by a number of different healthcare professionals. Normally patients remain fully clothed during a treatment session. It typically lasts about an hour. A practitioner will generally take details of a client's health before giving a treatment. Depending on the condition being treated, one treatment or a series of treatments may be recommended.

Clinical bottom line
Benefits
😕 *Unknown effectiveness*
- Dementia: not enough data available.
- Fibromyalgia: pain reduction yet not enough data available.

Risks
- *Contraindications:* phlebitis, deep vein thrombosis, burns, skin infections, eczema, open wounds, bone fractures, advanced osteoporosis.
- *Precautions/warnings:* cancer, myocardial infarction, osteoporosis, pregnancy.
- *Adverse effects:* rare. Serious adverse events such as jugular vein thrombosis, stroke and peripheral nerve damage have been reported. Mild to moderate pain during application of pressure is reported by most patients.

Conclusions
- No convincing data available to suggest that shiatsu is effective for any condition
- Adverse events are on record
- The risk–benefit balance fails to be positive

Further reading

Beresford-Cooke C. Shiatsu Theory and Practice: A Comprehensive Text for the Student and Professional. Edinburgh: Churchill Livingstone, 2003.
Shiatsu Society UK. http://www.shiatsusociety.org/

Spiritual healing

Definition
The use of spiritual means in treating disease. Interaction between a healer and a patient with the intention of generating improvements or a cure of the illness.

Concept
Healers believe they channel 'energy' (e.g. of cosmic or divine origin) into patients which helps the body to heal itself. The concept is not supported by scientific plausibility.

Related techniques
Therapeutic touch, Reiki, intercessory prayer, distant healing, Johrei, faith healing, laying on of hands, psychic healing, paranormal healing.

Treatment
Many different approaches of spiritual healing exist. Typically the healer moves their hands at a distance over the patient's body detecting areas of concern and transmits 'energy' into the patient's body which allegedly enhances self-healing. A session may last 30–60 minutes. Typically weekly sessions are prescribed. A series of treatments may consist of 6–10 sessions, which may be repeated regularly.

Clinical bottom line
Benefits
😐 *Unknown effectiveness*
- Johrei healing: scarce and unconvincing evidence for any condition.
- Reiki: the evidence is insufficient to suggest that it is an effective treatment for any condition.
- Therapeutic touch: no convincing evidence of effectiveness for any condition.

😟 *Unlikely to be beneficial:*
- Intercessory prayer: unlikely to be beneficial for any condition.
- Therapeutic touch: unlikely to be beneficial for promoting wound healing.

Risks
- *Contraindications:* psychiatric illness.
- *Precautions/warnings:* none known.
- *Adverse effects:* belief in supernatural 'energy' could undermine rational thought.
- *Interactions:* none known.

Conclusions

- Spiritual healing and all related techniques have not been convincingly demonstrated to be effective beyond placebo
- Few risks are on record
- The risk–benefit balance fails to be positive

Further reading

Jonas WB, Crawford C (eds). *Healing, Intention, and Energy Medicine*. Edinburgh: Churchill Living-stone, 2003.

Roberts L, Ahmed I, Hall S. Intercessory prayer for the alleviation of ill health. *Cochrane Database Syst Rev* 2007; **1**:CD000368.

National Federation of Spiritual Healers. http://www.nfsh.org.uk/

Static magnets

Definition

Magnets produce energy in the form of magnetic fields. Two main types of magnets can be distinguished. First, static or permanent magnets with a magnetic field that is unchanging and generated by the spin of electrons of the materials itself. Second, electromagnets with a magnetic field that is generated only when an electric current is applied. The magnetic field of the latter can be oscillating while the former is constant.

Concept

The majority of magnets marketed for self-treatment to consumers for health purposes are static magnets with varying strengths, typically between 30–500 mTesla. Magnets have been incorporated into arm and leg wraps, belts, mattress pads, necklaces, shoe inserts, and bracelets. They are usually made from iron, steel, or alloys and marketed for a wide range of diseases and conditions, including pain. None of the theories or claims explaining how static magnets might work have been conclusively proven. It is, however, conceivable that magnets might increase the temperature of the area of the body to which they are applied and some experiments suggest that it might have effects on cell function.

Related techniques

Electromagnetic field therapy.

Treatment

Static magnets are usually bought and used by patients directly, often without consulting a healthcare professional. Typically, the magnets are placed on the skin or placed inside clothing with close contact to the body. Depending on the condition, treatment with static magnets may vary and lasts for up to days or weeks of continuous or interrupted use.

Clinical bottom line
Benefits

☹ *Unknown effectiveness*

- Carpal tunnel syndrome: not more effective than placebo yet not enough data available.
- Depression: symptomatic effects in patients on antidepressants yet not enough data available.
- Facial paralysis: may improve facial tone but not enough data available.
- Fibromyalgia: may reduce pain yet not enough data available.
- Shoulder pain: may reduce frozen shoulder pain but not enough data available.
- Insomnia: improvement of quality and quantity of sleep, not enough data available.
- Knee pain, chronic: may reduce pain and enhance physical function, not enough data available.
- Neuropathy: reduction in pain and other symptoms, not enough data available.
- Osteoarthritis: encouraging yet conflicting data.

- Pelvic pain, chronic: not enough data available.
- Post polio, pain reduction: not enough data available.
- Primary dysmenorrhoea, pain reduction: not enough data available.
- Rheumatoid arthritis, pain: not enough data available.

🔯 *Likely to be ineffective or harmful*

- Breast cancer, hot flushes: likely to be ineffective.
- Delayed onset muscle soreness: likely to be ineffective.
- Ischemia, peripheral: likely to be ineffective.
- Low back pain, chronic: likely to be ineffective.
- Plantar heel pain: no evidence of effectiveness for insoles.

Risks

- *Contraindications:* pregnancy and lactation, pacemakers, insulin pumps.
- *Precautions/warnings:* wounds, acute sprains, inflammation.
- *Adverse effects:* generally considered to be safe, adverse effects are rare but reddening of the skin on the area of application has been observed.

Conclusions

- Insufficient data available to suggest that static magnets are effective for any condition
- Adverse events are rare
- The risk–benefit balance fails to be positive for any condition

Further reading

National Center for Complementary and Alternative Medicine. Questions and answers about using magnets to treat pain. *J Pain Palliat Care Pharmacother* 2005; **19**:59–72.

Tai chi

Definition

Rooted in ancient Chinese philosophy and martial arts, Tai chi is a system of movements and postures used to enhance mental and physical health. (pronounced /tie chee/).

Concept

Tai chi is based on the principles of the two opposing life forces, yin and yang, and is influenced by Confucian and Buddhist philosophy. Ill health is viewed as an imbalance between yin and yang. It is comprised of a series of postures linked by gentle and graceful movements. The slow movements between different postures that are normally held for a short period of time are physical stimuli with effects on the cardiovascular and muscular systems.

Related techniques

Qigong (pronounced /chee gong/).

Treatment

Tai chi is usually taught in classes of 5–10 or more. The student should maintain a level of concentration and not be distracted by external influences. The movements are performed simultaneously by the group responding to advice and corrections by the teacher. Tai chi is a lifelong endeavour and regular practice is essential in achieving beneficial effects. Daily practice is ideal but at least twice-weekly exercise is recommended.

Clinical bottom line

Benefits

😃 *Likely to be beneficial*
- Elderly patients: seems to improve physical performance and fear of falling.
- Hypertension: may reduce blood pressure yet data not fully convincing.
- Rheumatoid arthritis: range of motion outcomes of ankle plantar flexion, no detrimental effects on disease activity.

😐 *Unknown effectiveness*
- Anxiety: anxiolytic activity of regular tai chi reported but not enough data available.
- Cancer: may improve psychological and physiological symptoms but data not convincing.
- Chronic heart failure: increases in distance walked and quality of life yet more data required.
- Elderly patients: balance control, flexibility in patients with chronic conditions yet more data required.
- Falls: may improve balance and reduce falls yet trials are methodologically weak.
- Headache, tension-type: may improve headache status and quality of life measures yet not enough data available.
- Herpes zoster: increase in varicella zoster specific cell-mediated immunity but not enough data available.

- Osteoarthritis: may improve pain and function yet not enough data available.
- Postmenopausal women: retardation of bone loss yet more data required.

Risks

- *Contraindications:* largely based on common sense (e.g. severe osteoporosis, severe heart conditions, acute back pain, knee problems, sprains and fractures). Usually it can be safely practised during pregnancy and lactation.
- *Precautions/warnings:* before starting tai chi older individuals should be carefully examined for any of the above or other contraindications.
- *Adverse effects:* adverse effects are rare, but may include delayed-onset muscle soreness, pulled ligaments or ankle sprains.

Conclusions

- Seems helpful in rheumatoid arthritis, hypertension, and in physical performance of the elderly; it appears that these effects are similar to those of other physical exercise
- Only mild and infrequent adverse events
- Risk–benefit balance for the above conditions likely to be positive

Table 3.10 Systematic up-to-date reviews where tai chi has been found to be likely to be beneficial

Condition	Source	No. of trials/ patients	Original conclusion
Fear of falling	*J Am Geriatr Soc* 2007; **55**:603–15	N=3/n=441	Limited but fairly consistent findings in trials of higher methodological quality showed that home-based exercise and fall-related multifactorial programs and community-based tai chi delivered in group format have been effective in reducing fear of falling in community-living older people
Rheumatoid arthritis	*Cochrane Database Syst Rev* 2004; **3**: CD004849	N=4/n=206	The results suggest tai chi does not exacerbate symptoms of rheumatoid arthritis. In addition, tai chi has statistically significant benefits on lower extremity range of motion, in particular ankle range of motion

Further reading

Burke DT, Al-Adawi S, Lee YT, Audette J. Martial arts as sport and therapy. *J Sports Med Phys Fitness* 2007; **47**:96–102.
Taoist Tai Chi Society of Great Britain. http://www.taoist-tai-chi-gb.org/

Traditional Chinese medicine

Definition

Traditional Chinese medicine (TCM) is a diagnostic and therapeutic system based on complex (philosophical) theories, e.g. yin and yang theory and five-element theory. It is used as an umbrella term for approaches developed in ancient China, e.g. acupuncture, herbal medicines, tui-na (massage, pronounced /twi-na/), tai chi (pronounced /tie-chee/), diet.

Concept

According to TCM philosophy, health of an individual is maintained through the balance of yin and yang as well as non-disrupted flow and sufficient supply of vital energy called qi (pronounced /chee/), within the meridians. Disease is regarded as the result of imbalance of yin and yang or a blockage of vital energy.

Related techniques

Acupuncture, Chinese herbal medicine, tai chi, tui-na.

Treatment

TCM diagnostic methods include four aspects: observation (e.g. tongue, complexion), listening (may include smelling), asking questions (includes taking medical histories), and taking pulse. Treatment is based on the identification of particular patterns through the information gathered from the above techniques and tailored to the individual. One session may last 30–60 minutes. Depending on the nature of the condition, a treatment series may consist of 6–20 sessions. Often preventative treatments are encouraged.

Clinical bottom line

Benefits

In principle, the whole system of TCM could be tested by comparing outcomes with those of conventional medicine in a controlled clinical trial. Such global tests are, however, currently unavailable. Instead different defined modalities (e.g. acupuncture, herbal medicines or tai chi) have been submitted to clinical trials. The results of such investigations are reported in the respective chapters.

Risks

Generally speaking TCM has been associated with a range of risks; 📖 see respective chapters.
- *Contraindications:* depends on precise modality used.
- *Precautions/warnings:* depends on precise modality used.
- *Adverse effects:* depends on precise modality used.
- *Interactions:* depends on precise modality used.

Conclusions

- As a whole system, TCM has not been adequately tested for efficacy
- TCM is not devoid of risks, some are serious
- Risk–benefit balance is best evaluated according to specific modalities (📖 see respective chapters)

Further reading

Maciocia G. *The Foundations of Chinese Medicine* (2nd Edn). Edinburgh: Churchill Livingstone, 2005.

Yoga

Definition

Ancient Indian practice involving postural exercises, breathing control, and meditation.

Concept

The range of techniques is believed to increase the body's vital energy (prana). It leads to a relaxation response, a reduction of sympathetic drive. Breathing exercises may increase lung capacity. The totality of these measures can increase wellbeing.

Related techniques

Meditation, mind–body therapies.

Treatment

Yoga is best learnt under supervision of an experienced yoga teacher to avoid harm. Yoga classes take about 60–90 minutes and should be attended regularly. Yoga is, in many respects, a lifestyle regimen. Optimally, it should be followed regularly on a daily basis.

Clinical bottom line

Benefits

🙂 *Likely to be beneficial*

- Depression: encouraging data for symptom reduction.
- Hypertension: data are encouraging but not fully compelling.
- Normalization of cardiovascular risk factors such as stress, lack of physical activity, overweight: in conjunction with conventional treatments.

😐 *Unknown effectiveness*

- Attention deficit/hyperactivity disorder: not enough data available.
- Anxiety, stress management: contradictory results.
- Asthma: data contradictory.
- Back pain, pain and function: not enough data available.
- Cancer, palliation, fatigue, quality of life: not enough data available.
- Carpal tunnel syndrome: not enough data available.
- Diabetes, metabolic control: not enough data available.
- Drug dependence, methadone maintenance therapy: not enough data available.
- Epilepsy: may reduce seizure frequency yet not enough data available.
- Hot flushes, menopause: not enough data available.
- Hypercholesterolaemia: may cause a small reduction total cholesterol levels but data conflicting.
- Insomnia, sleep quality: not enough data available.
- Irritable bowel syndrome: not enough data available.
- Multiple sclerosis, symptom control, fatigue: not enough data available.
- Obsessive compulsive disorder: not enough data available.
- Osteoarthritis, pain, function: not enough data available.
- Pancreatitis, quality of life: not enough data available.
- Tuberculosis, dyspnoea: not enough data available.
- Visual discomfort after computer work: not enough data available.

✖ *Likely to be ineffective or harmful*
- Cognitive function in elderly people: trials fail to demonstrate effectiveness.
- Tinnitus: trials fail to demonstrate effectiveness.

Risks
- *Contraindications:* pregnancy (extreme posture), mental illness (meditation).
- *Precautions/warnings:* musculoskeletal injuries through overstretching joints.
- *Adverse effects:* drowsiness, one case of pneumothorax reported.
- *Interactions:* possibility of additive effects, e.g. with antihypertensives.

Conclusions

- Likely effective as an adjuvant treatment for normalizing several cardiovascular risk factors including hypertension and for depression
- Good safety record
- For cardiovascular risk reduction, hypertension and depression the risk–benefit balance is likely to be positive

Further reading

Coulter D. *Anatomy of Hatha Yoga: A Manual for Students, Teachers and Practitioners*. Delhi: Motilal Banarsidass, 2004.
The British Wheel of Yoga. http://www.bwy.org.uk/

Complementary medicines

African plum (*Prunus africana*)

Profile

Origin

African plum (*Prunus africana*, formerly *Pygeum africanum*) is a tree native to the mountainous regions of Sub-Saharan Africa and the Islands of Madagascar, Sao Tome, Fernando Po, and Grand Comore. The collection of mature bark to provide the raw material for its medicinal use has resulted in the species becoming endangered.

Main constituents

Sterols (beta-sitosterol), triterpenes. The active constituents have not been identified.

Presumed pharmacologic action

Anti-inflammatory, antiproliferative effects on fibroblasts. The mechanism of action is not known.

Commonly used dosage

100mg standardized extract daily.

Clinical bottom line

Benefits

:☺: *Beneficial*

- Benign prostatic hyperplasia: improves urinary symptoms and flow measures.

Table 4.1 Systematic up-to-date review where African plum has been found to be beneficial

Condition	Source	No. of trials/ patients	Original conclusion
Benign prostatic hyperplasia	*Cochrane Database Syst Rev* 2002; **1**:CD001044	N=18/n=1562	A standardized preparation of *P. africanum* may be a useful treatment option for men with lower urinary symptoms consistent with benign prostatic hyperplasia

Risks

- *Contraindications:* pregnancy and lactation.
- *Precautions/warnings:* no long-term safety data available.
- *Adverse effects:* nausea, abdominal pain.
- *Interactions:* may positively interact with 5 alpha-reductase inhibitors, saw palmetto or stinging nettle extracts.

Conclusions

- Best evidence suggests beneficial effects for treating benign prostatic hyperplasia
- Mild gastrointestinal adverse events have been reported
- The risk–benefit ratio for benign prostatic hyperplasia is positive

Further reading

Boulbes D, Soustelle L, Costa P et al. Pygeum africanum extract inhibits proliferation of human cultured prostatic fibroblasts and myofibroblasts. *BJU Int* 2006; **98**:1106–13.

Aloe (*Aloe vera*)

Profile
Origin
A cactus-like plant which grows in hot, dry climates. *Aloe vera* gel is made of mucilaginous tissue from the centre of the leaf. *Aloe vera* latex (also sap or aloes) is produced from the peripheral bundle sheath cells.

Main constituents
The gel contains several polysaccharides. The latex contains aloin, anthra-quinones, barbaloine, and glycosides.

Presumed pharmacologic action
- *Gel:* antimicrobial, anti-inflammatory, moisturizing, antipruritic.
- *Latex:* laxative, hypoglycaemic, hypolipo-proteinaemic.

Commonly used dosage
- *Gel*: applied liberally to the skin as needed.
- *Latex* (orally): common laxative dose is 100–200mg daily or 50mg taken in the evening.

Clinical bottom line
Benefits

😃 *Likely to be beneficial*
- Blood glucose: oral intake might reduce blood glucose and blood lipid levels.
- Herpes genitalis: topical application, best results for *Aloe vera* cream.

😐 *Unknown effectiveness*
- Constipation: may increase the frequency of bowel movements but not enough data available.
- Psoriasis vulgaris: data scarce and conflicting.
- Ulcerative colitis: oral intake, preliminary positive results for oral intake in mild-to-moderate ulcerative colitis but not enough data available.
- Wound healing, topical application: data conflicting.

😕 *Unlikely to be beneficial*
- Irritable bowel syndrome: no evidence of benefit in refractory secondary care patients.

🔯 *Likely to be ineffective or harmful*
- Oral mucositis: not effective in cancer patients receiving treatment.
- Radiation-induced skin reactions in cancer patients: no protective effects.
- Sunburn: ineffective in prevention and treatment.

Risks
- *Contraindications:* pregnancy, as aloe latex can induce abortions and stimulate menstruation; lactation; known allergy to plants from the *Liliaceae* family; intestinal obstruction; acute intestinal inflammation; ulcers; and haemorrhoids.

- *Precautions/warnings:* reflex stimulation of uterus could theoretically cause abortion in pregnant women. Should not be injected as this has been associated with serious complications and death. Use cautiously in patients with diabetes or glucose intolerance.
- *Adverse effects:* allergic skin reactions, damage to intestinal mucosa, delayed healing of deep wounds, red discolouration of urine, intestinal pain, diarrhoea, fluid or electrolyte loss.
- *Interactions:* increased effects of antiarrhythmics, cardiac glycosides, diuretics and steroids.

Conclusions

- Encouraging but not fully compelling evidence exists for blood glucose and lipid level control as well as genital herpes
- Topical use has few risks while oral administration is associated with considerable risks
- The risk–benefit balance is likely to be positive for genital herpes but is not convincingly positive for the control of blood glucose and lipid levels

Further reading

Boudreau MD, Beland FA. An evaluation of the biological and toxicological properties of *Aloe barbadensis* (Miller), *Aloe vera*. *Environ Sci Health C Environ Carcinog Ecotoxicol Rev* 2006; **24**:103–54.

Andrographis paniculata

Profile

Origin
Plant of the *Acanthaceae* family, native to Asia. Cultivated in many parts of the world. Leaf and rhizome are used for medicinal purposes. Used traditionally in Ayurvedic medicine.

Main constituents
Andrographolide, deoxyandrographolide, other diterpenes.

Presumed pharmacologic action
Immunostimulant, antibacterial, hepatoprotective, hypotensive.

Commonly used dosage
200–400mg extract standardized to 4–6mg andrographolide per day.

Clinical bottom line

Benefits
:😀: *Beneficial*
- Upper respiratory tract infections: may improve symptoms.

😑 *Unknown effectiveness*
- Other infections such as AIDS/HIV: not enough data available.

Table 4.2 Systematic up-to-date reviews where *Andrographis paniculata* has been found beneficial

Treatment	Source	No. of trials/ patients	Original conclusion
Upper respiratory tract infection	*Planta Medica* 2004; **70**:293–96	N=7/n=896	A. paniculata is superior to placebo in alleviating the subjective symptoms of uncomplicated upper respiratory tract infection.
Upper respiratory tract infection	*J Clin Pharm Ther* 2004; **29**:37–45	N=3/n=433	A. paniculata extract alone or in combination with A. senticosus extract may be more effective than placebo and may be an appropriate alternative treatment of uncompli-cated acute upper respiratory tract infection.

Risks
- *Contraindications:* pregnancy and lactation.
- *Precautions/warnings:* traditionally used as an abortificient.
- *Adverse effects:* allergic reactions, fatigue.
- *Interactions:* anti-platelet drugs, immunosuppressants, anti-hypertensives.

Conclusions

- Effective for symptomatic treatment of uncomplicated upper respiratory tract infections
- Relatively safe
- The risk–benefit balance for upper respiratory tract infections is positive

Further reading

Kligler B, Ulbricht C, Basch E et al. Andrographis paniculata for the treatment of upper respiratory infection: a systematic review by the natural standard research collaboration. *Explore (NY)* 2006; **2**:25–9.

Arnica (*Arnica montana*)

Profile

Origin
A perennial herbaceous plant native to the mountainous regions of Europe. The Latin name *Arnica* means 'lamb's skin' referring to its soft, hairy leaves. Preparations are made from the flowering heads.

Main constituents
Sesquiterpene lactones (helenalin), volatile oil, flavonoids.

Presumed pharmacologic action
Anti-inflammatory, antimicrobial.

Commonly used dosage
- *Homeopathic arnica, tincture*: 1:5, 45% application of 2–4mL.
- *Homeopathic arnica, poultice*: 2–3g arnica covered with 150mL hot water and strained after 10 minutes.

Clinical bottom line

Benefits

😕 *Unknown effectiveness*
- Muscle soreness after exercise: homeopathic arnica, data conflicting.
- Osteoarthritis: herbal tincture, may improve pain and function in hand osteoarthritis but not enough data available.
- Postoperative pain, swelling and bruising: homeopathic arnica, data conflicting.
- Tonsillectomy: homeopathic arnica, pain reduction but not enough data available.
- Traumatic injuries: homeopathic arnica, data inconclusive.

Risks
- *Contraindications:* pregnancy and lactation.
- *Precautions/warnings:* toxic by mouth unless extremely diluted (homeopathic preparations). Safe use for more than 2 weeks has not been well-studied. Avoid using topical arnica on open wounds or near the eyes and mouth. Theoretically arnica may increase the risk of bleeding: organ failure may occur from high doses.
- *Adverse effects:* non-homeopathic preparations or low homeopathic potencies: allergies, stomach discomfort, nausea and vomiting, liver and kidney damage, skin rashes, eczema, or lesions in the mouth. Possibly muscle weakness, organ damage, coma, and death. Irregular heart rhythms, rapid heartbeat, high blood pressure, or failure of the heart to beat may occur when arnica is taken by mouth, especially in large doses.
- *Interactions:* anticoagulants or antiplatelet drugs.

Conclusions

- There is no convincing evidence for any indication
- Only safe if used in highly diluted doses (orally) or short-term on unbroken skin (topically); otherwise considerable risks
- The risk–benefit balance fails to be positive

Further reading

Ludtke R, Hacke D. On the effectiveness of the homeopathic remedy Arnica montana. *Wien Med Wochenschr* 2005; **155**:482–90.

Artichoke (*Cynara scolymus*)

Profile
Origin
A herbaceous perennial. Avoid confusion with Jerusalem artichoke (*Helianthus tuberosa* L.), which is a species of sunflower. The leaves are used medicinally.

Main constituents
Flavonoids, phenolic acids, sesquiterpene lactones.

Presumed pharmacologic action
Hepatostimulating, diuretic, lipid lowering, carminative, antiemetic, choleretic. Indirect inhibitory effects at the level of HMG-CoA reductase. Cynarine (1.5-di-caffeoyl-D-quinic acid) or the flavonoid luteolin may be one of the principal active components.

Commonly used dosage
0.5–1.92g of dry extract daily in divided doses.

Clinical bottom line
Benefits

😊 *Likely to be beneficial*
- Hypercholesterolaemia: may reduce cholesterol levels but the evidence is not entirely compelling.
- Non-ulcer dyspepsia: may improve symptoms.

😐 *Unknown effectiveness*
- Irritable bowel syndrome: not enough data available.

☹ *Unlikely to be beneficial*
- Alcohol-induced hangover: not more effective than placebo.

Risks
- *Contraindications:* allergies to artichoke and related species (*Asteraceae* or *Compositae*), obstruction of bile duct. Pregnancy and lactation.
- *Precautions/warnings:* gallstones, bile duct obstruction.
- *Adverse effects:* flatulence, allergic reactions.
- *Interactions:* none known.

Conclusions
- Data suggest that it may be effective for hypercholesterolaemia and for symptom improvement in non-ulcer-dyspepsia, yet the data are not entirely convincing
- Adverse events such as flatulence and allergic reactions have been reported
- The risk–benefit balance is not convincingly positive for any condition but likely to be positive for the above two conditions

Avocado-soybean unsaponifiables

Profile

Origin

Made out of that fraction of soy and avocado oil (3.1) which cannot be turned into soap.

Main constituents

Not clearly defined.

Presumed pharmacologic action

Inhibition of interleukin–1 synthesis, stimulation of collagen synthesis, anti-inflammatory, anabolic.

Commonly used dosage

300–600mg per day.

Clinical bottom line

Benefits

☺ Likely to be beneficial

- Osteoarthritis: symptom control but the trial data are not entirely uniform

Table 4.3 Systematic up-to-date review where avocado-soybean unsaponifiables (ASU) have been found likely to be beneficial

Treatment	Source	No. of trials/ patients	Original conclusion
Osteoarthritis	*Clin Rheumatol* 2003; **22**:285–8	N=4/n=750	The majority of the rigorous trial data … suggest that ASU is effective for the symptomatic treatment of osteoarthritis

Risks

- *Contraindications:* pregnancy and lactation.
- *Precautions/warnings:* none known.
- *Adverse effects:* none known.
- *Interactions:* none known.

Conclusions

- Some, but not all, evidence suggests effectiveness for osteoarthritis
- No known risks
- The risk–benefit balance might be positive for osteoarthritis

Bilberry (*Vaccinium myrtillus*)

Profile
Origin
A deciduous dwarf shrub of the *Ericaceae* family native to Europe, North America, and Northern Asia. Close relative of blueberry (*V. corymbosum*). The fruits are mainly used for medicinal purposes.

Main constituents
Anthocyanosides, tannins, flavonoids.

Presumed pharmacologic action
Improves microcirculation, inhibition of prostacyclin synthesis, astringent, antioxidant, antiplatelet, anti-inflammatory, and antioedema activity.

Commonly used dosage
- *Orally:* 80–480mg daily in divided doses.
- *Topically:* berries are applied as a 10% decoction.

Clinical bottom line
Benefits

😐 *Unknown effectiveness*
- Chronic venous insufficiency: improvements in symptom severity but data scarce with methodological limitations.
- Degenerative eye disorders: not enough data available.
- Dysmenorrhoea: encouraging results but not enough data available.

🗶 *Likely to be ineffective or harmful*
- Night vision: likely to be ineffective.

Risks
- *Contraindications:* theoretical risk of increased bleeding in those with bleeding disorders or in patients taking anticoagulants. Theoretical risk of hypoglycaemia in diabetics and patients taking hypoglycaemic medications.
- *Precautions/warnings:* limit doses to those recommended as toxicity may theoretically occur at higher doses. Leaves may be toxic when ingested.
- *Adverse effects:* mild gastrointestinal complaints.
- *Interactions:* Theoretical risk of interaction with NSAIDs, drugs and herbs with anticoagulant activity, antiplatelet agents, and hypoglycaemics.

Conclusions
- Effectiveness has not been established for any condition
- Generally considered safe when consumed in recommended doses but risk of interactions exist
- The risk–benefit balance fails to be positive for any condition

Black cohosh (*Actaea racemosa*)

Profile

Origin
A shrub native to North America: member of the buttercup family. Dried root and rhizome are used medicinally.

Main constituents
27-deoxyactein, actein, cimicifugoside, salicylic acid.

Presumed pharmacologic action
Oestrogen-like activity, hypotensive, anti-inflammatory.

Commonly used dosage
80–160mg of standardized extract in divided dosages, providing 4–8mg of 27-deoxyactein per day.

Clinical bottom line

Benefits

⊕⊖ *Trade off between benefits and harms*
- Menopause: may reduce hot flushes and depressive symptoms.

☹ *Unknown effectiveness*
- Cancer, palliation: hot flushes, data conflicting.
- Menopausal symptoms, other than hot flushes or depression: not enough data available.

Risks
- *Contraindications:* pregnancy and lactation.
- *Precautions/warnings:* patients treated for hypertension.
- *Adverse effects:* in rare cases liver damage has been associated with black cohosh.
- *Interactions:* hypotensives, hepatotoxic drugs.

Conclusions

- Likely to be effective for treating menopausal hot flushes and depressive symptoms
- Adverse events are rare but have been associated with liver damage
- The risk–benefit balance for treating hot flushes and depressive symptoms in menopausal women can be positive but regular liver function tests are required

Further reading

Carroll DG. Nonhormonal therapies for hot flashes in menopause. *Am Fam Physician* 2006; **73**:457–64.

Butcher's broom (*Ruscus aculeatus*)

Profile

Origin

A lignified plant growing wild in woods and undergrowth in all of Europe. Rhizome and roots are used for medicinal purposes.

Main constituents

Steroid saponins (ruscogenin and neoruscogenin), benzofuranes, flavonoids, essential oil.

Presumed pharmacologic action

The steroidal saponin constituents produce vasoconstrictive effects by direct activation of alpha-adrenergic receptors.

Commonly used dosage

Oral: 300–600mg of dried extract.
Topical: 4–6g of cream containing 64–96mg of extract.

Clinical bottom line

Benefits

:☻: *Beneficial*

- Chronic venous insufficiency: a combination of butcher's broom root, hesperidin methyl chalcone and ascorbic acid (Cyclo 3 Fort®) reduces severity of symptoms.

☻ *Unknown effectiveness*

- Chronic venous insufficiency: monopreparation, not enough data available.

Table 4.4 Systematic up-to-date review where butcher's broom has been found to be beneficial

Condition	Source	No. of trials/ patients	Original conclusion
Chronic venous insufficiency	*Int Angiol* 2003; **22**:250–62	N=25/n=10246	In patients with chronic venous insufficiency Cyclo 3 Fort® significantly reduces the severity of symptoms compared to placebo

Risks

- *Contraindications:* pregnancy and lactation.
- *Precautions/warnings:* none known.
- *Adverse effects:* can cause gastrointestinal disorders and in rare cases nausea.
- *Interactions:* none known.

Conclusions

- There is evidence of effectiveness for a combination product, Cyclo 3 Fort®, in chronic venous insufficiency but the role of butcher's broom on its own is unclear
- Only mild risks are on record
- The risk–benefit balance for the combination product Cyclo 3 Fort® is positive

Butterbur (*Petasites hybridus*)

Profile

Origin

A herbaceous perennial plant in the daisy family (Asteraceae), native to Europe, northern Asia and parts of North America. The plant has been traditionally used for stomach cramps, whooping cough, and asthma, and now is growing in popularity for treating allergic rhinitis. Leaves, rhizome and roots are used medicinally.

Main constituents

Petasin, isopetasin.

Pharmacologic action

Antispasmodic and anti-inflammatory properties. May inhibit the biosynthesis of cysteinyl leukotrienes and decrease nasal levels of histamine and cysteinyl leukotrienes.

Commonly used dosage

100–150mg root extract.

Clinical bottom line

Benefits

☺ *Likely to be beneficial*
- Migraine, prevention: seems to reduce frequency of attacks.
- Seasonal allergic rhinitis: seems to reduce symptom severity.

☹ *Unknown effectiveness*
- Atopic asthma: may improve force expiratory volume and symptoms yet not enough data available.

Table 4.5 Systematic up-to-date reviews where butterbur has been found likely to be beneficial

Condition	Source	No. of trials/ patients	Original conclusion
Allergic rhinitis	*Ann Allergy, Asthma Immunology* 2007 (in press)	N=6/n=720	There is encouraging evidence suggesting that *P. hybridus* may be an effective herbal treatment for intermittent allergic rhinitis
Migraine	*Phytomedicine* 2006; **13**:743–6	N=2/n=293	There is to date moderate evidence of effectiveness for a 3–4 months daily treatment with 150mg *Petasites* root extract Petadolex® in the prophylaxis of migraine

Risks
- *Contraindications:* liver damage, pregnancy, and lactation.
- *Precautions/warnings:* may contain hepatotoxic pyrrolizidine alkaloids: should only be taken when prepared by a reputable laboratory; long-term safety has not been studied.
- *Adverse effects:* gastrointestinal complaints.
- *Interactions:* none reported.

Conclusions
- Data suggests that butterbur is likely to be beneficial for migraine prevention and intermittent allergic rhinitis. The evidence is however not entirely convincing for any condition
- Gastrointestinal adverse events may occur
- The risk–benefit fails to be convincingly positive for any condition but is likely to be positive for the above two conditions

Further reading
Giles M, Ulbricht C, Khalsa KP *et al*. National Standard Research Collaboration. Butterbur: an evidence-based systematic review by the natural standard research collaboration. *J Herb Pharmacother* 2005; **5**:119–43.

Cannabis (*Cannabis sativa*)

Profile
Origin
The genus Cannabis includes the three species, *Cannabis sativa* L., *Cannabis indica* Lam., and *Cannabis ruderalis* Janisch, which are indigenous to central Asia. The term hemp usually refers to varieties of Cannabis cultivated for its abundance of fiber and non-drug use. Cannabis plants produce a group of chemicals—cannabinoids—which have mental and physical effects when consumed. Due to widespread illegal use of cannabis as a recreational drug its legal or licensed use in medicine is a controversial issue in most countries.

Main constituents
Delta-9-tetrahydrocannabinol.

Presumed pharmacologic action
Antiemetic, antispasmodic, analgesic.

Commonly used dosage
- *Oral*: dronabinol, the prescription product for chemotherapy-induced nausea and vomiting is used in doses of 5–15mg/m^2 body surface every 2–4 hours.
- *Inhalation*: 65–195mg for smoking.

Clinical bottom line
Benefits

😃 *Likely to be beneficial*
- Multiple sclerosis: seems to reduce pain and spasticity but data not fully convincing.

😐 *Unknown effectiveness*
- Brachial plexus root convulsion: may improve pain and sleep quality yet not enough data available.
- Multiple sclerosis: may reduce the number of incontinence episodes yet not enough data available.
- Neuropathy, HIV-associated: may reduce pain yet not enough data available.
- Rheumatoid arthritis: pain on movement and resting pain yet not enough data available.

😟 *Unlikely to be beneficial*
- Multiple sclerosis: seems unlikely to be beneficial in reducing tremor.
- Parkinson's disease: seems unlikely to improve dyskinesia.

🔀 *Likely to be ineffective or harmful*
- Cancer-related anorexia-cachexia syndrome: seems ineffective in improving appetite and quality of life.

Risks
- *Contraindications:* pregnancy and lactation.
- *Precautions/warnings:* potential to be addictive.

- *Adverse effects:* dizziness, sleepiness, fatigue, bad taste. Intoxicating doses impair reaction time, motor coordination, and visual perceptions; can produce panic reactions, hallucinations, flashbacks, depression, and other emotional disturbances.
- *Interactions:* barbiturates, fluoxetine or disulfiram, theophylline. Additive or synergistic effects with amphetamines, anticholinergics, antihistamines, cocaine, hypnotics, psychomimetics, sedatives, and sympathomimetics.

Conclusions

- Cannabis extract is likely to be beneficial for reducing pain and spasticity in multiple sclerosis. The evidence is however not fully convincing
- A number of adverse events are on record. In controlled conditions using high quality products these may be manageable
- The risk–benefit ratio for reducing pain and spasticity in patients with multiple sclerosis is not entirely positive

Further reading

Mills RJ, Yap L, Young CA. Treatment for ataxia in multiple sclerosis. *Cochrane Database Syst Rev* 2007; **1**:CD005029.

Chamomile (*Matricaria recutita*)

Profile

Origin

An annual herb belonging to the *Asteraceae* family. Flowerheads are used medicinally.

Main constituents

Capric acid, coumarins, flavonoids (apigenin), spiroethers, tannins, terpenoid volatile oils (chamazulene, alpha bisabolol).

Presumed pharmacologic action

Antibacterial, anti-inflammatory, antispasmodic.

Commonly used dosage

- *Liquid extract:* 1–4mL (1:1 in 45% alcohol) 3 times daily.
- *Dried flowers:* 3g in 150mL hot water 3 times daily.

Clinical bottom line

Benefits

😃 *Likely to be beneficial*

- Diarrhoea, acute, unspecific childhood diarrhoea: a combination preparation seems to reduce duration and stool frequency.
- Dyspepsia, functional: data suggest effectiveness of a combination preparation (STW5).

😐 *Unknown effectiveness*

- Anxiety: not enough data available.
- Common cold: symptom improvement after steam inhalation yet not enough data available.
- Eczema: topical preparation, not enough data available.
- Irradiation skin damage, in breast cancer patients: not enough data available.
- Irritable bowel syndrome: not enough data available.
- Skin aging: encouraging results of a combination preparation yet not enough data available.

🙁 *Likely to be ineffective or harmful*

- Postoperative sore throat, hoarseness: preparation as a mouthwash seems ineffective in preventing the condition.
- Stomatitis: preparation as a mouthwash seems ineffective.

Risks

- *Contraindications:* pregnancy and lactation.
- *Precautions/warnings:* known sensitivity to other members of the *Asteraceae* family (e.g. asters, chrysanthemums, sunflowers), asthma, or other allergic conditions.
- *Adverse effects:* allergic reactions, vomiting.
- *Interactions:* theoretically, the effects of anticoagulants and central nervous system depressants could be potentiated and the level of drugs metabolized by cytochrome P450 3A4 could be increased.

Conclusions

- The evidence is likely beneficial for a combination preparation in acute unspecific childhood diarrhoea and for another combination preparation (STW5) in patients with functional dyspepsia
- There is the risk of allergic reactions
- Given the risk of allergic reactions and the few data from rigorous clinical trials, the evidence is not entirely convincing of whether the benefits outweigh the risks

Further reading

McKay DL, Blumberg JB. A review of the bioactivity and potential health benefits of chamomile tea (*Matricaria recutita* L.). *Phytother Res* 2006; **20**:519–30.

Chaste tree (*Vitex agnus-castus*)

Profile

Origin
Member of the *Verbenaceae* family. Native to the Mediterranean region and western Asia. Root, bark, and fruit are used for medicinal purposes.

Main constituents
Diterpens, flavonoids, iridoids, linoleic acid.

Presumed pharmacologic action
Hypoprolactinaemic, dopaminergic, anti-inflammatory, antiandrogenic, anti-microbial.

Commonly used dosage
40mg of standardized extract per day.

Clinical bottom line

Benefits

🙂 *Likely to be beneficial*
- Mastalgia: reduces pain in cyclical mastalgia.

😐 *Unknown effectiveness*
- Female infertility: not enough data available.
- Luteal deficiency: not enough data available.
- Premenstrual syndrome, symptom control: best trial data contradictory.

✖ *Likely to be ineffective or harmful*
- Bust-enhancing treatment: likely to be ineffective.

Risks
- *Contraindications:* pregnancy and lactation.
- *Precautions/warnings:* changes to the menstrual cycle are possible
- *Adverse effects:* usually mild and transient, e.g. acne, allergic reactions, gastrointestinal problems.
- *Interactions:* theoretically it could interact with a range of hormonal therapies.

Conclusions

- Chaste tree extracts are likely to relieve pain from cyclical mastalgia
- No serious risks are known
- The risk–benefit balance is likely to be positive for cyclical mastalgia

Further reading
Wuttke W, Jarry H, Christoffel V *et al.* Chaste tree (Vitex agnus-castus)—pharmacology and clinical indications. *Phytomedicine* 2003; **10**:348–57.

.

Chilli (*Capsicum* spp)

Profile
Origin
Chilli peppers and their various cultivars originate in the Americas. The substances that give chilli peppers their intensity when ingested or applied topically are capsaicin and several related chemicals, collectively called capsaicinoids. They are widely used in medicine and cuisine and are a rich source of vitamin C and provitamin A.

Main constituents
Capsaicin (8-methyl-N-vanillyl-6-nonenamide).

Pharmacologic action
Analgesic.

Commonly used dosage
3–4 times daily topically. Cream or plaster containing 0.025–0.075% capsaicin applied in the area of pain.

Clinical bottom line
Benefits
Data refer to applications of topical capsaicin if not otherwise stated.

:☺: *Beneficial*
- Musculoskeletal pain: reduces pain.
- Neuropathic pain, chronic: reduces pain of various causes.

☺ *Likely to be beneficial*
- Back pain: seems to reduce pain.
- Neuralgia, postherpetic: seems to reduce pain.
- Pruritus: seems to reduce pruritus of various causes.
- Psoriasis: seems to reduce itching, scaling, and erythema.

☻ *Unknown effectiveness*
- Abdominal hysterectomy: may reduce postoperative opioid requirements yet not enough data available.
- Cluster headache: may reduce pain yet not enough data available.
- Complex regional pain syndrome: may reduce pain but too few data available.
- Dyspepsia, functional: ingestion of red pepper powder may improve epigastric pain, nausea and sensation of fullness but too few data available.
- Inguinal hernia: may reduce postoperative opioid requirements in children yet not enough data available.
- Neurogenic hyperreflexic bladder: intravesical capsaicin may improve urodynamic symptoms.
- Neuropathic cancer pain: may be effective for pain reduction yet not enough data available.
- Osteoarthritis: may be effective for pain reduction yet not enough data available.
- Overweight/obesity: may reduce body fat mass yet not enough data available.

- Post-mastectomy syndrome: may reduce pain yet not enough data available.
- Vulvar vestibulitis: may reduce pain yet not enough data available.

😣 *Unlikely to be beneficial*
- Bladder pain, severe: intravesical capsaicin, unlikely to be beneficial.
- Temporomandibular pain: unlikely to be beneficial for pain reduction.

💀 *Likely to be ineffective or harmful*
- HIV-related peripheral neuropathy: ineffective in relieving pain.

Table 4.6 Systematic up-to-date review where capsaicin has been found to be beneficial

Condition	Source	No. of trials/ patients	Original conclusion
Musculoskeletal pain; neuropathic pain	*BMJ* 2004; **328**:991	N=3/n=368; N=6/n=656	Although topically applied capsaicin has moderate to poor efficacy in the treatment of chronic musculoskeletal or neuropathic pain, it may be useful as an adjunct or sole therapy for a small number of patients who are unresponsive to, or intolerant of, other treatments

Risks
- *Contraindications:* pregnancy and lactation.
- *Precautions/warnings:* inflammatory skin conditions and wounds, do not use near the eyes or on sensitive skin.
- *Adverse effects:* skin irritation, burning sensation, gastrointestinal complaints.
- *Interactions:* none.

Conclusions

- Capsaicin, the main constituent of chilli, is beneficial for reducing musculoskeletal and neuropathic pain and likely to be beneficial for several other conditions
- Adverse events with topical use appear to be mild
- The risk–benefit ratio for musculoskeletal and neuropathic pain is positive and likely to be positive for back pain, neuralgia, pruritus and psoriasis

Further reading

Pingle SC, Matta JA, Ahern GP. Capsaicin receptor: TRPV1 a promiscuous TRP channel. *Handb Exp Pharmacol* 2007; **179**:155–71.

Final report on the safety assessment of capsicum annuum extract, capsicum annuum fruit extract, capsicum annuum resin, capsicum annuum fruit powder, capsicum frutescens fruit, capsicum frutescens fruit extract, capsicum frutescens resin, and capsaicin. *Int J Toxicol.* 2007; **26**:3–106.

Chitosan

Profile

Origin

Shells of crustacean and various fungi.

Main constituents

Chitosan: N-deacetylated form of chitin, a hydrophilic positively charged polysaccharide.

Presumed pharmacologic action

Hypocholesterolaemic, hypolipidaemic, fat-binding (in vitro), haemostatic.

Commonly used dosage

2g of deacetylated chitin biopolymer daily in divided doses.

Clinical bottom line

Benefits

☺ *Likely to be beneficial*
- Hypercholesterolaemia: may reduce total and LDL cholesterol.

☹ *Unknown effectiveness*
- Bleeding control: may have positive effects on bleeding time as compared to manual compression yet not enough data available.
- Dental plaque formation: some positive findings but not enough data available.

✗ *Unlikely to be beneficial*
- Body weight: effects are minimal and unlikely to be of clinical significance.

Risks

- *Contraindications*: pregnancy and lactation.
- *Precautions/warnings*: lack of relevant safety data relating to effects in women taking oral contraceptives.
- *Adverse effects*: constipation, flatulence, diarrhoea, nausea.
- *Interactions*: may slow the absorption of oral contraceptives.

Conclusions

- Best evidence suggests that there is no indication which is supported by convincing evidence of effectiveness but it is likely to be effective in reducing total and LDL cholesterol levels
- A number of adverse events have been reported particularly constipation, flatulence, diarrhoea and nausea
- The risk–benefit balance is likely to be positive for hypercholesterolaemia

Further reading

Ni Mhurchu C, Dunshea-Mooij CA, Bennett D, Rodgers A. Chitosan for overweight or obesity. *Cochrane Database Syst Rev* 2005; **3**:CD003892.

Shi C, Zhu Y, Ran X *et al.* Therapeutic potential of chitosan and its derivatives in regenerative medicine. *J Surg Res* 2006; **133**:185–92.

Chondroitin

Profile

Origin

Bovine tracheal cartilage.

Main constituents

Glycosaminoglycans, e.g. chondroitin-4-sulphate, chondroitin-6-sulphate, N-acetylgalactosamine.

Presumed pharmacologic action

Rebuilds cartilage, anti-inflammatory, inhibition of leukocyte elastase and hyaluronidase, increases synovial viscosity.

Commonly used dosage

800–1200mg chondroitin sulphate.

Clinical bottom line

Benefits

:☺: *Beneficial*

- Osteoarthritis, pain and function: even though not all studies agree, the totality of the evidence indicates efficacy. Chondroitin may even prevent joint space narrowing in osteoarthritis.

☻ *Unknown effectiveness*

- Overactive bladder: preliminary results have suggested positive symptomatic effects.

Risks

- *Contraindications:* pregnancy and lactation.
- *Precautions/warnings:* bleeding abnormalities, asthma.
- *Adverse effects:* dyspepsia, headache, nausea.
- *Interactions:* anticoagulants.

Conclusions

- Good evidence for efficacy in osteoarthritis for chondroitin sulphate but small effect size
- Only minor risks have been reported
- The risk–benefit balance seems to be positive
- The value of chondroitin relative to conventional treatments is not clear

Further reading

Bjordal JM, Klovning A, Ljunggren AE, Slordal L. Short-term efficacy of pharmacotherapeutic interventions in osteoarthritic knee pain: A meta-analysis of randomized placebo-controlled trials. *Eur J Pain* 2007; **11**:125–38.

Chromium

Profile

Origin

A chemical element with atomic number 24 in the periodic table. Small quantities of chromium are needed for glucose utilization in normal health. As a nutritional supplement chromium picolinate ($Cr(C_6H_4NO_2)_3$, the chromium (III) salt of picolinic acid, is used. It is claimed to aid body development in athletes, help lose body weight, and reduce insulin resistance in diabetics.

Main constituents

Chromium picolinate.

Presumed pharmacologic action

Antidiabetic, body fat reducing.

Commonly used dosage

200–1000mcg.

Clinical bottom line

Benefits

😊 *Likely to be beneficial*

- Diabetes, type 2: reductions in hyperglycaemia and hyperinsulinaemia.

😐 *Unknown effectiveness*

- Depression: not enough data available.
- Hypertension: may reduce HDL levels in patients taking beta-blockers.

☹ *Unlikely to be beneficial*

- Athletes: unlikely to be beneficial for increasing exercise performance or muscular strength.
- Body weight reduction: unlikely to be beneficial.
- Healthy persons: unlikely to have effects on lipid levels, insulin sensitivity or body composition.
- Overweight/obesity: effects, if any, are of debatable clinical relevance.

Table 4.7 Systematic up-to-date reviews where chromium has been found to be beneficial or likely to be beneficial

Treatment	Source	No. of trials/ patients	Original conclusion
Diabetes, type 2	*Diabetes Technol Ther* 2006; **8**:677–87	N=15/n=1690	Pooled data from studies using chromium picolinate supplementation for type 2 diabetes mellitus subjects show substantial reductions in hyperglycemia and hyperinsulinemia [...]

Risks
- *Contraindications:* pregnancy and lactation.
- *Precautions/warnings:* care should be taken not to overdose.
- *Adverse effects:* rhabdomyolysis, renal impairment, exanthematous pustulosis.
- *Interactions:* none known.

Conclusions

- Chromium picolinate is likely to be beneficial for hyperglycemia and hyperinsulinemia in type 2 diabetic patients
- Risks are on record
- The risk–benefit balance fails to be convincingly positive for any indication
- Until further data become available other treatment approaches should be preferred for type 2 diabetic patients

Further reading

A scientific review: the role of chromium in insulin resistance. Diabetes Educ 2004; (Suppl):2–14.

Coenzyme Q10

Profile

Origin

Produced by the human body. Present in most cells, the highest concentrations are found in the heart, liver, kidneys and pancreas. Synthesized in large quantities for the food supplement market by fermenting sugar beets and sugar cane with special strains of yeast.

Main constituents

Ubiquinones.

Presumed pharmacologic action

Participates on the cellular level in the electron transfer within the oxidative respiration chain in the mitochondria, thus preventing adenosine triphosphate depletion as well as oxidant and ischaemic cellular damage. Membrane stabilizer, free radical scavenger, and co-factor in many metabolic processes.

Commonly used dosage

50–300mg of coenzyme Q10 daily, higher dosages of up to 3000mg daily have been used.

Clinical bottom line

Benefits

😊 *Likely to be beneficial*
- Hypertension: reductions of blood pressure when administered with other antihypertensives.

😐 *Unknown effectiveness*
- Aerobic exercise: data conflicting.
- Cancer, tolerability of treatments: some protection against cardiotoxicity and liver toxicity but data scarce and methodologically weak.
- Cardiac surgery: improves mitochondrial function before cardiac surgery but not enough data available.
- Chronic renal failure: improves renal functions but not enough data available.
- Diabetes: might lower HbA1c and blood pressure but not enough data available.
- Heart failure: data conflicting.
- Migraine: reduces attack-frequency, headache-days and days-with-nausea but not enough data available.
- Muscular dystrophy: improved physical performance but not enough data available.
- Myocardial protection: data conflicting.
- Parkinson's disease: slowing progressive deterioration of function with high dosage of coenzyme Q10 (1200mg daily) but not enough data available.

😞 *Unlikely to be beneficial*
- Hypercholesterolaemia: no reductions of total cholesterol reported.

✖ *Likely to be ineffective or harmful*
- Cocaine dependence: no positive effects.
- Huntington's disease: no positive effects.
- Periodontal disease: no positive effects.

Table 4.8 Systematic up-to-date review where coenzyme Q10 has been found likely to be beneficial

Treatment	Source	No. of trials/ patients	Original conclusion
Hypertension	*BioFactors* 2003; **18**:91–100	N=8/n=397	Being devoid of significant side effects CoQ10 may have a role as an adjunct or alternative to conventional agents in the treatment of hypertension

Risks
- *Contraindications:* pregnancy and lactation, known allergy (probably rare).
- *Precautions/warnings:* excessive exercise should be avoided.
- *Adverse effects:* diarrhoea and other gastrointestinal complaints such as nausea, vomiting, occur in less than 1% of patients.
- *Interactions:* theoretically decreases the effects of warfarin: HMG-CoA reductase inhibitors might decrease coenzyme Q10 levels: additional blood pressure lowering effects when used with antihypertensive drugs.

Conclusions

- Encouraging evidence for lowering blood pressure when administered with other antihypertensives
- Associated with only few risks
- For hypertension the risk–benefit balance is likely to be positive

Cranberry (*Vaccinium macrocarpon*)

Profile

Origin
Evergreen shrubs which grow in most temperate climates. Berries are used for medicinal purposes.

Main constituents
Catechin, flavone glycosides, fructose, organic acids, proanthocyanidins, vitamin C.

Presumed pharmacologic action
Probably inhibiting the adhesion of bacteria to the uroepithelial surface by proanthycanidin and fructose. It does not, however, seem to have the ability to release bacteria which are already adhered to the urinary tract epithelial cells.

Commonly used dosage
There are no clear dosing guidelines: recommended doses range from 90–480mL of cranberry juice twice daily; 300–400mg of standardized extract twice daily.

Clinical bottom line

Benefits

☺ *Likely to be beneficial*
- Urinary tract infections, prevention: best results reported for women.

☻ *Unknown effectiveness*
- Urinary stone risk factors: mixed effects on urinary stone forming properties, not enough data available.
- Urinary tract infections: treatment, not enough data available.

☒ *Likely to be ineffective or harmful*
- Neurogenic bladder secondary to spinal cord injury: ineffective in preventing urinary tract infections.
- Prostate cancer: no efficacy for symptoms.

Table 4.9 Systematic up-to-date review where cranberry has been found likely to be beneficial

Condition	Source	No. of trials/ patients	Original conclusion
Urinary tract infection, prevention	*Cochrane Database Syst Rev* 2004; **2**: CD001321	N=7/n=604	Cranberry juice may decrease the number of symptomatic UTIs over a 12 month period in women

Risks
- *Contraindications:* pregnancy and lactation.
- *Precautions/warnings:* should not be taken as a substitute for antibiotic treatment, diabetics should consider high sugar content of the juice.
- *Adverse effects:* none known.
- *Overdose:* doses of over 3L daily may cause gastrointestinal distress and diarrhoea. Toxicity in infants and young children.
- *Interactions:* could theoretically enhance the elimination of drugs excreted in urine or increase effects of some antibiotics in the urinary tract. Potentially between cranberry and warfarin.

Conclusions

- There is some evidence that cranberry juice may be useful in the prevention of urinary tract infections in women but its effects in other populations (e.g. the elderly, children) are unclear
- Cranberry is relatively safe if consumed in recommended doses
- The risk–benefit balance for cranberry in preventing urinary tract infections in women is likely to be positive

Devil's claw (*Harpagophytum procumbens*)

Profile
Origin
A plant growing wild in South Africa that has unique looking fruits covered with claw-like hooks. Tuberous roots used for medicinal purposes.

Main constituents
Harpagoside.

Presumed pharmacologic action
Anti-inflammatory, analgesic, negative chronotropic, positive inotropic, antiarrhythmic.

Commonly used dosage
400–500mg of dried extract 3 times daily.

Clinical bottom line
Benefits

:☺: *Beneficial*
- Back pain: best results with aqueous extract at a daily dose equivalent of 50mg harpagoside.
- Osteoarthritis: harpagophytum powder at 60mg harpagoside in the treatment of osteoarthritis of the spine, hip and knee.

Table 4.10 Systematic up-to-date review where devil's claw has been found to be beneficial

Condition	Source	No. of trials/ patients	Original conclusion
Osteoarthritis and low back pain	*BMC Complement Altern Med* 2004; 4:13	N=12/n=1105	There is moderate evidence of effectiveness for the use of a *Harpagophytum* powder at 60mg harpagoside in the treatment of osteoarthritis of the spine, hip and knee … Strong evidence exists for the use of an aqueous *Harpagophytum* extract at a daily dose equivalent of 50mg harpagoside in the treatment of acute exacerbations of chronic non-specific low-back pain

Risks

- *Contraindications:* pregnancy (uterus stimulating effects) and lactation, gastric or duodenal ulcer, gallstones.
- *Precautions/warnings:* insufficient reliable data about topical or long-term use available, might lower blood sugar levels.
- *Adverse effects:* gastrointestinal symptoms, allergic skin reactions.
- *Interactions:* may increase anticoagulation effects of warfarin, theoretically interacts with cardiac drugs.

Conclusions

- Positive evidence for its effectiveness in musculoskeletal pain associated with back pain and osteoarthritis
- Only mild adverse events on record
- The risk–benefit balance is positive for back pain and osteoarthritis
- Comparative trials report it to be equally effective as conventional treatment options, e.g. NSAIDs

Further reading

Brendler T, Gruenwald J, Ulbricht C et al. Devil's claw (*Harpagophytum procumbens* DC): an evidence-based systematic review by the Natural Standard Research Collaboration. *J Herb Pharmacother* 2006; **6**:89–126.

Dong quai (*Angelica sinensis*)

Profile

Origin

A plant popular in most Asian medical traditions. The roots and leafs are used for medicinal purposes. Dong quai is employed mostly in herbal combination products or prescriptions.

Main constituents

Ligustilide, ferulic acid, safrole.

Presumed pharmacologic action

Oestrogenic, anticoagulant, platelet inhibitor.

Commonly used dosage

1–5g of root or equivalent daily.

Clinical bottom line

Benefits

🙂 *Unknown effectiveness*
- Breast enlargement: not enough data available.

😧 *Unlikely to be beneficial*
- Menopause, symptom control: does not reduce menopausal symptoms, no oestrogenic effects.

Risks
- *Contraindications:* none known.
- *Precautions/warnings:* pregnancy, lactation, photosensitivity.
- *Adverse effects:* allergic reactions, safrole may be carcinogenic, gastro-intestinal symptoms.
- *Interactions:* anticoagulants, anti-arrhythmic drugs.

Conclusions

- The use of dong quai is not supported by good evidence for any indication
- Several serious adverse effects are on record
- The risk–benefit balance fails to be positive

Echinacea (*Echinacea* spp)

Profile
Origin
One of the most popular herbal remedies on the US and European markets. Three different species are mainly used for medicinal purposes: roots of *E. angustifolia* and *E. pallida*, roots and other parts of *E. purpurea*.

Main constituents
Alkylamides, caffeic acid derivatives, glycoproteins, ketoalkenes/ketoalkynes (*E. pallida* only), polysaccharides.

Presumed pharmacologic action
Modulates cellular and hormonal immune defence, local anaesthetic, anti-inflammatory, activation of adrenal cortex, antiviral, antifungal, free radical scavenger.

Commonly used dosage
- *Capsules of powered herb:* 500–1000mg, 3 times daily.
- *Juice:* 6–9mL daily in divided doses.
- *Tincture (1:5):* 0.75–1.5mL 2–5 times daily.
- *Tea:* 4g of echinacea in one cup of water.

Clinical bottom line
Benefits
Echinacea preparations tested in clinical trials differ greatly.

😊 *Likely to be beneficial*
- Common cold, treatment: some evidence that preparations based on the aerial parts of *E. purpurea* might be effective for the early treatment of colds in adults but results are not fully consistent.

☒ *Likely to be ineffective or harmful*
- Common cold: prevention, no effect over placebo.
- General immune response: not effective in stimulating immune response in healthy young men.
- Herpes genitalis: not effective for treatment.

Table 4.11 Systematic up-to-date reviews where echinacea has been found likely to be beneficial

Condition	Source	No. of trials/ patients	Original conclusion
Common cold	*Cochrane Database Syst Rev* 2006; **1**:CD000530	N=7/n=1158	There is some evidence that preparations based on the aerial parts of *Echinacea purpurea* might be effective for the early treatment of colds in adults but results are not fully consistent

tus (*Eucalyptus globulus*)

re than 700 species of Eucalyptus, mostly native to Australia
calypti are evergreen. As in other members of the myrtle
otus leaves are covered with oil glands. The oil is readily
d and can be used for cleaning, deodorizing, and in food
especially sweets, cough drops, and decongestants.

ents
eucalyptol), tannins, phenolic acids, flavonoids.

ic action
ti-inflammatory, expectorant.

sed dosage
,8 cineol): 600mg daily in capsules.

ttom line

effectiveness
nay reduce oral steroid medication yet not enough data

ivity: seems to have no effect when combined with
nt oil.
mation: may reduce plaque formation yet not enough data

lemon eucalyptus extract (Citriodiol®) may be useful as
ellent.

cations: allergies to eucalyptus species or any constituents
nflammatory conditions of the gastrointestinal tract, liver
regnancy and lactation.
s/*warnings:* eucalyptus oil, as a volatile oil, contains constitu-
are toxic if ingested internally. Infants and young children.
ffects: nausea, vomiting, diarrhoea in rare cases.
ns: none known.

ions
ggest that there is no convincing evidence that eucalyptus is
al for any condition
verse events are on record
<–benefit fails to be positive for any condition

Risks
- *Contraindications:* pregnancy and lactation.
- *Precautions/warnings:* patients suffering from progressive systemic diseases (e.g. AIDS/HIV, multiple sclerosis); drug-free intervals are recommended when used for more than 8 weeks.
- *Adverse effects:* allergic reactions, rash in children, gastrointestinal complaints.
- *Interactions:* could theoretically decrease effects of immunosuppressants.

Conclusions
- Some encouraging yet not compelling evidence relating to the early treatment of the common cold with *Echinacea purpurea* exists
- No serious risks have been reported, adverse events in adults seem to be rare
- The risk–benefit balance for *E. purpurea* in the early treatment of the common cold is likely to be positive

Further reading
Barnes J, Anderson LA, Gibbons S, Phillipson JD. Echinacea species *Echinacea angustifolia* (DC.) Hell., *Echinacea pallida* (Nutt.) Nutt.,*Echinacea purpurea* (L.) Moench): a review of their chemistry, pharmacology and clinical properties. *J Pharm Pharmacol* 2005; **57**:929–54.
Huntley AL, Thompson Coon J, Ernst E. The safety of herbal medicinal products derived from Echinacea species: a systematic review. *Drug Saf* 2005; **28**:387–400.
Linde K, Barrett B, Wolkart K *et al*. Echinacea for preventing and treating the common cold. *Cochrane Database Syst Rev* 2006; **1**:CD000530.

Ephedra (*Ephedra sinica*, ma huang)

Profile

Origin
Small perennial evergreen shrub frequently used in traditional Chinese Medicine. Aerial parts are used for medicinal purposes.

Main constituents
Ephedrine and other stimulants.

Presumed pharmacologic action
Sympathomimetic, increase in metabolic rate.

Commonly used dosage
15–90mg ephedra alkaloids calculated as ephedrine per day.

Clinical bottom line

Benefits

⚖ *Trade off between benefits and harms*
- Weight loss, small effect is well-documented but considerable cardiovascular risks are recorded.

☹ *Unknown effectiveness*
- Aphrodisiac for women: not enough data available.
- Asthma: data insufficient.
- Hypercholesterolaemia: data insufficient.
- Increase of physical performance: data insufficient.

Table 4.12 Systematic up-to-date review where ephedra has been found to be beneficial

Condition	Source	No. of trials/patients	Original conclusion
Weight loss performance	*JAMA* 2003; **289**:1537–45	N=18/n=not available	Ephedra promotes modest short-term weight loss

Risks
- *Contraindications:* artheriosclerosis, hypertension, diabetes.
- *Precautions/warnings:* pregnancy and lactation.
- *Adverse effects:* dry mouth, insomnia, nervousness, myocardial infarction, palpitations, increased heart rate and blood pressure, increase of QT-interval, stroke.
- *Interactions:* other sympathomimetics, MOA-inhibitors, cardiovascular drugs, antidiabetics, steroids.

Conclusions
- A small reduction of body weigh
- The cardiovascular risks are con
- The risk–benefit balance fails to

Further reading
Andraws R, Chawla P, Brown DL. Cardiovascu
   review. *Prog Cardiovasc Dis* 2005; **47**:217–25.

Eucaly

Profile

Origin
There are m
Nearly all e
family, euca
steam distill
supplements

Main consti
Volatile oils

Pharmacolo
Antiseptic, a

Commonly
Eucalyptol (

Clinical b

Benefits

☹ *Unknow*
- Asthma:
  available.
- Pain sens
  peppern
- Plaque fe
  available
- Repellen
  insect re

Risks
- *Contrain*
  thereof,
  disease,
- *Precautio*
  ents tha
- *Adverse*
- *Interacti*

Conclu
- Data s
  benefi
- Rare a
- The ri

Evening primrose (*Oenothera biennis*)

Profile

Origin
Evening primrose (*Onagraceae* family) is native to North America. For medicinal purposes the oil from seeds is used.

Main constituents
Cis-linoleic acid (about 70%), cis-gamma linoleic acid (about 9%).

Presumed pharmacologic action
Anti-inflammatory.

Commonly used dosage
3–4g per day (neuralgia), 6–8g per day (eczema).

Clinical bottom line

Benefits

😐 *Unknown effectiveness*
- Chronic fatigue syndrome: date scarce and contradictory.
- Diabetic neuropathy, pain: not enough data available.
- Uraemic pruritus: not enough data available.

🗶 *Likely to be ineffective or harmful*
- Asthma, lung function, symptom control: likely to be ineffective.
- Attention deficit disorder: not an effective treatment.
- Eczema: initial positive studies were superseded by more rigorous negative trials.
- Menopause, bone density, hot flushes: likely to be ineffective.
- Obesity, weight control: likely to be ineffective.
- Premenstrual syndrome, symptom control, mastalgia: likely to be ineffective.
- Psoriasis, remission rate: likely to be ineffective.
- Schizophrenia: not enough data available.
- Sjögren's syndrome, fatigue: likely to be ineffective.
- Ulcerative colitis: may improve stool consistency but not enough data available.

Risks
- *Contraindications:* pregnancy, lactation.
- *Precautions/warnings:* epilepsy.
- *Adverse effects:* headache, gastrointestinal symptoms.
- *Interactions:* anti-inflammatory drugs, corticosteroids, beta-blockers, antipsychotics, anticoagulants.

Conclusions

- No sound evidence of benefit for any condition
- Some risks are known but serious adverse effects seem rare
- The risk–benefit balance fails to be positive

Fennel (*Foeniculum vulgare*)

Profile

Origin
The fruit and the oil of the fennel plant which is indigenous to the Mediterranean region are used.

Main constituents
Anethole, fenchone, estragole.

Presumed pharmacologic action
Promotes gastrointestinal motility, antispasmodic, mucociliary activity, allergenic.

Commonly used dosage
- Dried fruit: 5–7g.
- Infusion: 1–2g of fruit or seed in 150mL water, 3 times daily.
- 0.1–0.6mL oil.

Clinical bottom line

Benefits

😐 *Unknown effectiveness*
- Colic in infants: promising results for fennel seed oil but not enough data available.
- Dysmenorrhoea: similar results as with mefenamic acid for pain but only few data available.
- Hirsutism: topical fennel extract shows encouraging results in idiopathic hirsutism but not enough data available.
- Menopause: preliminary data suggest a reduction in hot flushes.

Risks
- *Contraindications:* pregnancy (emmenagogue effects) and lactation.
- *Precautions/warnings:* the constituent estragole is a procarcinogen, safety of long-term use is unknown.
- *Adverse effects:* allergic reactions affecting the skin and respiratory system, photodermatitis.
- *Interactions:* might reduce ciprofloxacin bioavailability.

Conclusions

- There is no compelling evidence of effectiveness for fennel for any condition
- Relatively safe when used short-term orally in food amounts but not long-term or in pregnancy
- The risk–benefit balance fails to be positive for any indication

Fenugreek (*Trigonella foenum-graecum*)

Profile

Origin
Commonly used in India as a condiment. Long history of medicinal use. Seeds are employed for medicinal purposes.

Main constituents
Coumarins, saponins.

Presumed pharmacologic action
Anti-diabetic, cholesterol-lowering, cholagogue, anti-inflammatory, galactogogue.

Commonly used dosage
10–15g powdered seeds per day.

Clinical bottom line

Benefits

😕 *Unknown effectiveness*
- Diabetes: might improve blood glucose and triglyceride levels but not enough data available.
- Hypercholesterolaemia: may reduce total, LDL, and HDL cholesterol but not enough data available.
- Hypertriglyceridaemia: not enough data available.

Risks
- *Contraindications:* none known.
- *Precautions/warnings:* pregnancy, lactation.
- *Adverse effects:* gastrointestinal symptoms, allergic reactions.
- *Interactions:* anticoagulants, antidiabetics.

Conclusions

- Some encouraging evidence for diabetes and dyslipoproteinanaemias but it is far from convincing
- No serious safety concerns are known
- The risk–benefit balance fails to be convincingly positive

Feverfew (*Tanacetum parthenium*)

Profile

Origin
Feverfew is a perennial plant native to Asia Minor.

Main constituents
Camphor, chrysanthenyl acetate and flavonoids. Parthenolide is thought to be the active principle.

Presumed pharmacologic action
Analgetic, anti-inflammatory, antithrombotic, cytotoxic, spasmolytic. Parthenolide may exert inhibiting effects on serotonin release by human platelets in vitro. Chrysanthenyl acetate may be important. It has been shown to inhibit prostaglandin synthesis in vitro and may possess analgesic properties.

Commonly used dosage
50–140mg of powdered or granulated dried leaf preparation daily in divided doses.

Clinical bottom line

Benefits

😐 *Unknown effectiveness*
- Migraine, prevention: data contradictory.

😕 *Unlikely to be beneficial*
- Rheumatoid arthritis: no relevant effects on clinical or laboratory parameters.

Risks
- *Contraindications:* pregnancy and lactation, hypersensitivity to members of the *Asteraceae* family.
- *Precautions/warnings:* should not be used for longer than 4 months due to the lack of long-term toxicity data.
- *Adverse effects:* allergic reactions, contact dermatitis, mouth ulceration and soreness, gastrointestinal complaints, 'post-feverfew syndrome' including rebound of migraine symptoms, anxiety, dizziness, insomnia, muscle and joint stiffness.
- *Interactions:* may potentiate the effects of anticoagulants.

Conclusions
- There is no convincing evidence for any condition
- Some but no serious adverse events have been reported
- The risk–benefit balance fails to be positive

Fish oil (omega-3 fatty acids)

Profile

Origin
Omega-3(n=3) fatty acids derived from oily fish.

Main constituents
Eicosapentaenoic acid (EPA) and docosahexaenoic acid (DHA).

Presumed pharmacologic action
Anti-inflammatory, inhibition of platelet aggregation, hypotensive, cholesterol-lowering, anti-coagulant, reduction of heart rate.

Commonly used dosage
Up to 3.8g EPA and 2g DHA per day.

Clinical bottom line

Benefits
Based on systematic reviews only.

😊 Beneficial
- Dyslipoproteinaemia: lowers triglyceride and increases HDL-levels.
- Hypertension: small effect on systolic and diastolic blood pressure.
- Rheumatoid arthritis: reduces tender joint count and morning stiffness.

😃 Likely to be beneficial
- Attention-deficit/hyperactivity disorder: most trials are positive.
- Cardiovascular disease (myocardial infarction, cardiac and sudden death, stroke): reduction of mortality.
- Crohn's disease: symptom control.
- Cystic fibrosis: symptomatic improvements.
- Intermittent claudication: positive effects on haemodynamic but not on clinical outcomes.
- Pregnancy: small effect on pregnancy duration and head circumference.
- Renitis pigmentosa: slowing of progression.
- Total mortality: supplementation is associated with longer life.

😐 Unknown effectiveness
- Asthma: not enough data available.
- Cancer cachexia: data contradictory.
- Childhood learning abilities: data methodologically weak.
- Cognitive function in healthy people: not enough data available.
- Dementia: cognitive function, some results are encouraging but totality of evidence inconclusive.
- Depression: small protective effect of EPA but evidence limited and heterogenous
- Kidney transplant, long-term outcome: data inconsistent.
- Macular degeneration: data methodologically weak.
- Pre-eclampsia, prevention: not enough data available.
- Schizophrenia: not enough data available.

✖ *Likely to be ineffective or harmful*
- Angina pectoris: no effect on symptoms.
- Atopic dermatitis: best studies fail to demonstrate effectiveness.
- Cancer prevention: (based largely on epidemiological data): data negative.
- Diabetes: no effects on glycaemic control.

Risks

- *Contraindications:* none known.
- *Precautions/warnings:* bleeding time may be marginally prolonged, some preparations may be contaminated by heavy metals.
- *Adverse effects:* allergic reactions, gastrointestinal symptoms.
- *Interactions:* anticoagulants.

Conclusions

- Fish oil supplementation is beneficial for dyslipoproteinaemia, hypertension, and rheumatoid arthritis and likely to be beneficial for a range of conditions
- Even though some risks are known these are usually small and manageable
- For the above-listed indications, the risk–benefit balance is positive

Further reading

Appleton KM, Hayward RC, Gunnell D *et al.* Effects of n-3 long-chain polyunsaturated fatty acids on depressed mood: systematic review of published trials. *Am J Clin Nutr* 2006; **84**:1308–16.

Hooper L, Thompson RL, Harrison RA *et al.* Risks and benefits of omega 3 fats for mortality, cardiovascular disease, and cancer: systematic review. *BMJ* 2006; **332**:752–60.

Lee S, Gura KM, Kim S *et al.* Current clinical applications of omega-6 and omega-3 fatty acids. *Nutr Clin Pract* 2006; **21**:323–41.

Flaxseed (*Linum usitatissimum*)

Profile

Origin

Flax is an annual plant which originated in India. The seeds and oil are used orally and topically.

Main constituents

- *Flaxseed*: fibre, mucilages, fatty oil, proteins, lignans.
- *Oil*: linolenic, linoleic and oleic acids.

Presumed pharmacologic action

- Flaxseed (not oil): antioxidant oestrogen receptor agonist/antagonist properties, laxative.
- Flaxseed and oil: lipid-lowering properties.

Commonly used dosage

- *Flaxseed*: up to 50g daily.
- *Oil*: 7g of alpha-linolic acid per 15mL, 15–30mL daily.
- *Liquid*: 1 tablespoon of the whole or bruised (not ground) seed with 150mL water up to 3 times daily.

Clinical bottom line

Benefits

😕 *Unknown effectiveness*

- Benign prostatic hyperplasia: not enough data available.
- Breast cancer, flaxseed (not oil): alters tumour biological markers but not enough data from human clinical trials available.
- Hypercholesterolaemia: results contradictory.
- Lupus nephritis, flaxseed (not oil): might lower serum creatinines but not enough data available.
- Menopausal symptoms: may help decrease mild menopausal complaints but no effect on hot flushes reported.

😟 *Unlikely to be beneficial*

- Rheumatoid arthritis.

Risks

- *Contraindications:* flaxseed (not oil): diarrhoea, irritable bowel syndrome, diverticulitis, inflammatory bowel disease; pregnancy (emmenagogue effects) and lactation.
- *Precautions/warnings:* might increase risk of prostate cancer; unripe flaxseed pods might be poisonous; large amounts of flaxseed (not oil) by mouth might cause obstruction of bowels; should be used cautiously in women with hormone-sensitive conditions, persons with diabetes or high triglyceride levels; oil must not be applied to open wounds or broken skin.
- *Adverse effects:* allergies.
- *Interactions:* may reduce the absorption of other medication, can theoretically increase the risk of bleeding.

Conclusions

- There is not enough evidence of effectiveness for any condition
- Several risks have been reported
- The risk–benefit balance fails to be positive for any condition

French maritime pine (*Pinus pinaster*)

Profile

Origin
The maritime pine (*Pinus pinaster*) is a tree native to the western Mediterranean region reaching a height of 20–35m. Pycnogenol® is a widely available water extract of the bark of French maritime pine.

Main constituents
Oligomeric proanthocyanidins, catechin, epicatechin, ferulic acid, caffeic acid, taxifolin.

Presumed pharmacologic action
Antioxidant, anti-inflammatory, reduction of capillary permeability.

Commonly used dosage
100–200mg daily of French maritime pine bark water extract.

Clinical bottom line

Benefits

🙂 *Unknown effectiveness*
- Asthma: may improve pulmonary function and asthma symptoms yet not enough data available.
- Attention deficit hyperactivity disorder: may improve symptoms but data contradictory.
- Diabetes, type 2: may lower HbA1c levels and may slow progression of diabetic retinopathy yet not enough data available.
- Gingival bleeding: may reduce bleeding time and dental plaque formation.
- Hypertension: may reduce the need for antihypertensive medication but not enough data available.
- Venous insufficiency, chronic: not enough data available.

Risks
- *Contraindications:* allergy to any part of *P. pinaster*, pregnancy and lactation.
- *Precautions/warnings:* may increase the risk of bleeding.
- *Adverse effects:* gastrointestinal complaints.
- *Interactions:* may interact with anti-diabetic medication.

Conclusions

- Data suggests no convincing evidence for any condition
- Few and mild adverse events are reported
- The risk–benefit ratio fails to be positive for any condition

Garlic (*Allium sativum*)

Profile

Origin
A member of the onion family *Alliaceae*. It has a long traditional use for culinary and medicinal purposes. For medicinal purposes bulbs are freeze dried or the oil is extracted.

Main constituents
Alliin which is converted to allicin.

Presumed pharmacologic action
Antimicrobial, antihypertensive, antidiabetic, antithrombotic, antimutagenic.

Commonly used dosage
- *Bulb:* 4g of fresh garlic daily.
- *Oil:* 8mg daily.

Clinical bottom line

Benefits

:☺: *Beneficial*
- Cancer, prevention: particularly gastrointestinal cancers.

☺ *Likely to be beneficial*
- Hypercholesterolaemia: effect is statistically significant but small and thus of debatable clinical relevance.

☻ *Unknown effectiveness*
- Arteriosclerosis, prevention: a range of single effects seem to act together.
- Common cold, prevention: not enough data available.
- Diabetes: might have a small effect on dyslipidaemia but not enough data available.
- Hair loss: as an adjunct topical treatment to corticosteroids but not enough data available.
- Hypertension: small effect on blood pressure control but data not convincing.
- Mosquito repellent: not enough data available.
- Peripheral arterial occlusive disease: improvement in pain-free walking distance but not enough data available.
- Pre-eclampsia: not enough data available.
- Rheumatoid arthritis: not enough data available.
- Tick bites, prevention: not enough data available.

Table 4.13 Systematic up-to-date review where garlic has been found likely to be beneficial

Treatment	Source	No. of trials/ patients	Original conclusion
Hypercholestero-laemia	*Phytopharmaka VII. Darmstadt: Steinkopff: 2002*	N=16/n=971	Garlic is superior to placebo but the effect is small

Risks
- *Contraindications:* pregnancy and lactation, peptic ulcer.
- *Precautions/warnings:* hypercoagulability.
- *Adverse effects:* bad breath, allergic reactions, heartburn, gastrointestinal symptoms.
- *Interactions:* anticoagulants, antidiabetics.

Conclusions

- Can be useful in the prevention of cancer (particularly gastrointestinal) and likely to be useful for hypercholesterolaemia
- Some risks are on record
- With adequate usage, risk–benefit balance can be positive for cancer prevention and is likely to be positive for hypercholesterolaemia
- Regular garlic intake is merely an adjunct to a conventional strategy of risk minimization

Further reading

Rahman K, Lowe GM. Garlic and cardiovascular disease: a critical review. *J Nutr* 2006; **136**:736S–40S.

Ginger (*Zingiber officinale*)

Profile

Origin

A perennial plant native to southern Asia. The rhizome is used medicinally.

Main constituents

Niacin, non-pungent substances, non-volatile pungent principles, starch, triglycerides, vitamins, and volatile oil.

Presumed pharmacologic action

Antiemetic, anti-inflammatory, positive inotropic, carminative, promotes secretion of saliva and gastric juices, cholagogue, inhibition of platelet aggregation.

Commonly used dosage

0.5–1g extract in divided doses or 1–4g dried powdered root daily.

Clinical bottom line

Benefits

☺: *Beneficial*

- Nausea/vomiting, postoperative: effective beyond placebo for this condition but effect might be of small clinical relevance.

⊕ *Trade off between benefits and harms*

- Nausea/vomiting, pregnancy-induced: frequency may be reduced, seems relatively safe but more comprehensive safety data required.

☻ *Unknown effectiveness*

- Motion sickness: earlier positive reports were corroborated but not enough data available.
- Nausea/vomiting, chemotherapy-induced: some positive effects were reported when compared with standard antiemetic drugs but not enough data available.
- Osteoarthritis: no convincing data for pain relief.

Table 4.14 Systematic up-to-date reviews where ginger has been found to be effective or likely to be effective

Condition	Source	No. of trials/ patients	Original conclusion
Postoperative nausea and vomiting	*Am J Obstet Gynecol* 2006; **194**:95–9	N=5/n=363	A fixed dose of at least 1g of ginger is more effective than placebo for the prevention of postoperative nausea and vomiting and postoperative vomiting
Nausea and vomiting in pregnancy	*Obstet Gynecol* 2005; **105**; 846–56	N=7/n=862	Ginger may be an effective treatment for nausea and vomiting in pregnancy

Risks

- *Contraindications:* pregnancy and lactation: a clinical review found no scientific or medical evidence for the contraindication of ginger during pregnancy; there is, however, a theoretical risk of congenital deformity in neonates. Allergy to members of the *Zingiberaceae* family.
- *Precautions/warnings:* children under 6 years of age; gallstones. Patients using anticoagulants, prior to surgery.
- *Adverse effects:* heartburn, belching, bloating, flatulence, nausea; mutagenic potential shown in vitro studies requires further systematic investigations.
- *Interactions:* increased effects of anticoagulants; may interfere with cardiac and antidiabetic therapy; may enhance the effects of central nervous system depressants.

Conclusions

- For treating postoperative nausea and vomiting best evidence suggests effectiveness whereas for pregnancy-induced nausea and vomiting the evidence is encouraging but not fully convincing. Due to the theoretical risk of congenital deformity in neonates it is contraindicated in this condition
- Allergies and interactions need to be considered
- The risk–benefit balance suggests that it is worthy of consideration for postoperative nausea and vomiting

Further reading

Chrubasik S, Pittler MH, Roufogalis BD. Zingiberis rhizoma: a comprehensive review on the ginger effect and efficacy profiles. *Phytomedicine* 2005; **12**:684–701.

Ginkgo (*Ginkgo biloba*)

Profile

Origin

The ginkgo tree is native to China, Korea, and Japan. It is the last remaining member of the Ginkgoaceae family. Leaves are used for medicinal purposes.

Main constituents

Bilobalide, ginkgolides, flavonoids.

Presumed pharmacologic action

Increase of microcirculatory blood flow, inhibition of platelet and erythrocyte aggregation, platelet-activating factor antagonism, free radical scavenging.

Commonly used dosage

- *Dementia and memory impairment:* 120–240mg of standardized leaf extract daily in divided doses.
- *Intermittent claudication, vertigo, tinnitus:* 120–160mg of standardized leaf extract daily in divided doses.

Clinical bottom line

Benefits

:☺: *Beneficial*

- Cognitive impairment and dementia: evidence of improvement in cognition and function.
- Peripheral arterial occlusive disease: modest increase in pain-free and maximal walking distance.

☺ *Likely to be beneficial*

- Hearing loss, sudden: encouraging effects have been reported but data not fully convincing.

☹ *Unknown effectiveness*

- Anxiety disorder: positive effects on Hamilton anxiety scale, further data required.
- Cancer, palliation: reduced limb heaviness in patients with lymphoedema after breast cancer treatment, yet not enough data available.
- Cognitive function, healthy people: evidence conflicting.
- Depression: no effects for winter depression yet not enough data available.
- Erectile dysfunction: not enough data available.
- Glaucoma, normal tension: effects have been reported but not enough data available.
- Macular degeneration: for preventing progression but not enough data available.
- Multiple sclerosis: some positive evidence for symptom severity, fatigue and functionality but not cognitive functions, not enough data available.
- Nephropathy, diabetic: not enough data available.
- Premenstrual syndrome: preliminary data for breast pain and nostalgia but more data required.
- Raynaud's syndrome: encouraging yet not enough data available.

- Schizophrenia: encouraging yet not enough data available.
- Stroke: may improve attention, reaction time, and short-term memory yet no convincing evidence available.
- Vitiligo: encouraging yet not enough data available.

🙁 *Unlikely to be beneficial*
- Drug dependency: unlikely to be beneficial for cocaine dependency.
- Hypertension: evidence is insufficient for treatment recommendations.
- Tinnitus: unlikely to be beneficial.

☒ *Likely to be ineffective or harmful*
- Acute mountain sickness, prevention: likely to be ineffective.
- Chronic venous insufficiency: likely to be ineffective in improving symptoms.
- Menopause: does not seem to reduce depression or anxiety in this population.
- Sexual dysfunction, antidepressant-induced: seems ineffective beyond placebo for this condition.

Table 4.15 Systematic up-to-date reviews where ginkgo has been found to be beneficial

Condition	Source	No. of trials/ patients	Original conclusion
Cognitive impairment and dementia	*Cochrane Database Syst Rev* 2002; **4**: CD003120	N=33/n=4247	Appears to be safe in use with no excess side effects compared with placebo. Overall there is promising evidence of improvement in cognition and function
Peripheral arterial occlusive disease	*Atherosclerosis* 2005; **181**:1–7	N=9/n=619	*G. biloba* extract seems more effective than placebo for patients with intermittent claudication

Risks
- *Contraindications:* pregnancy and lactation, hypersensitivity to *G. biloba*-containing preparations.
- *Precautions/warnings:* effects in children under 12 years are largely unknown.
- *Adverse effects:* gastrointestinal disturbances, diarrhoea, vomiting, allergic reactions, pruritus, headache, dizziness, epileptic seizures, Stevens–Johnson syndrome.
- *Interactions:* Possible potentiation of anticoagulants. It has been suggested that ginkgo at recommended doses does not affect clotting status, the pharmacokinetics, or pharmacodynamics of warfarin in healthy subjects. May have additive effects on antihypertensive drugs, or drugs used in the management of vascular erectile dysfunction.

Conclusions

- Ginkgo is beneficial for peripheral arterial occlusive disease, cognitive impairment, and dementia and likely to be beneficial for loss of hearing
- Gastrointestinal disturbances, allergic reactions, and pruritus are reported as adverse events
- The risk–benefit balance for peripheral arterial occlusive disease, cognitive impairment and dementia is positive and likely to be positive for loss of hearing

Further reading

Bent S, Goldberg H, Padula A, Avins AL. Spontaneous bleeding associated with Ginkgo biloba: a case report and systematic review of the literature. *J Gen Intern Med* 2005; **20**:657–61.

Dugoua JJ, Mills E, Perri D, Koren G. Safety and efficacy of ginkgo (*Ginkgo biloba*) during pregnancy and lactation. *Can J Clin Pharmacol* 2006; **13**:e277–84.

Ginseng, Asian (*Panax ginseng*)

Profile

Origin
A perennial herb native to the mountain forests of China and Korea.

Main constituents
Triterpene saponins known as ginsenosides or panaxosides.

Presumed pharmacologic action
Anti-inflammatory, antitumour, immunomodulatory, hypoglycaemic, smooth muscle relaxant and stimulatory.

Commonly used dosage
- *Extract*: 100mg of standardized extract (4% total ginsenosides) 2–3 times daily.
- *Root*: 0.5–2.0g of dry root daily in divided doses.

Clinical bottom line

Benefits
😊 *Likely to be beneficial*
- Erectile dysfunction: evidence is encouraging but not entirely convincing for penile rigidity, girth, and libido.

😐 *Unknown effectiveness*
- Cancer, palliation: positive effects in treating fatigue and on quality of life in patients receiving chemotherapy but not enough data available.
- Cancer, prevention: reductions in risk but not enough data available.
- Chronic heart failure: haemodynamic improvements have been suggested but not enough data available.
- Chronic obstructive pulmonary disease: might improve pulmonary function but not enough data available.
- Diabetes: improvements of fasting blood glucose levels and HbA1c but data scarce and contradictory.
- Hypertension: blood pressure normalizing effects but not enough data available.
- Upper respiratory tract infection: reduced frequency of colds and flu and increased immune activity but not enough data available.

😕 *Unlikely to be beneficial*
- Menopause: no improvement of quality of life, hot flushes or vaginal cytology.

🧿 *Likely to be ineffective of harmful*
- Alzheimer's disease: likely to be ineffective in improving somatic symptoms, depression and anxiety.
- Hypercholesterolaemia: likely to be ineffective.

Risks
- *Contraindications*: pregnancy and lactation.
- *Precautions/warnings*: hypertension, cardiovascular disease, hypotension, diabetes, patients receiving steroid therapy.

- *Adverse effects:* insomnia, excitability, anxiety, diarrhoea, vaginal bleeding, nosebleeds, mastalgia, increased libido, manic symptoms, skin rash, Stevens–Johnson syndrome, anaphylaxis.
- *Interactions:* monoamine oxidase inhibitors such as phenelzine may reduce the effects of warfarin, increased effects of hypoglycaemics.

Conclusions

- The effectiveness of Asian ginseng root extract is encouraging for erectile dysfunction but has not been established beyond reasonable doubt for any indication
- A number of adverse events and interactions have been reported including reduced effectiveness of warfarin
- The risk–benefit balance fails to be positive for any condition

Ginseng, Siberian (*Eleutherococcus senticosus*)

Profile

Origin

A slender shrub native to Siberia and northern China.

Main constituents

Eleutherosides (A–G), starch, vitamin A.

Presumed pharmacologic action

Antioxidant, antiproliferative, hypoglycaemic, immunostimulatory, inhibition of platelet aggregation.

Commonly used dosage

100–200mg of solid (20:1) extract daily in divided doses.

Clinical bottom line

Benefits

😐 *Unknown effectiveness*

- Healthy persons: some positive effects are reported for psychomotor performance and cognitive function but not enough data available.
- Herpes simplex type II infections: might improve severity, duration and frequency of attacks but not enough data available.
- Pneumonia, non-specific: some positive results for a combination preparation yet not enough data available.
- Upper respiratory tract infection: not enough data available.

😟 *Unlikely to be beneficial*

- Chronic fatigue syndrome: no improvements reported relative to placebo.

Risks

- *Contraindications:* pregnancy and lactation, hypertension, children under the age of 12 years.
- *Precautions/warnings:* premenopausal women, fever, mania, schizophrenia, asthma, diabetes, cardiac disorders.
- *Adverse effects:* dizziness, drowsiness, anxiety, irritability, hypertension, pericardial pain, tachycardia, extrasystoles, insomnia, headaches, mastalgia, diarrhoea.
- *Interactions:* may increase the effects of anxiolytic, sedative, antihyperglycaemic and antihyperglycaemic agents, may increase serum digoxin levels, may interact with cardiac, hypo- and hypertensive and anticoagulant agents, may inhibit cytochrome P450 1A2 and P450 2C9.

Conclusions

- The effectiveness of Siberian ginseng root extract is not established beyond reasonable doubt for any indication
- The possibility of adverse effects and drug interactions exists
- The reported risks may outweigh any potentially beneficial effects

Further reading

Buettner C, Yeh GY, Phillips RS et al. Systematic review of the effects of ginseng on cardiovascular risk factors. *Ann Pharmacother* 2006; **40**:83–95.

Palisin TE, Stacy JJ. Ginseng: is it in the root? *Curr Sports Med Rep* 2006; **5**:210–4.

Glucosamine

Profile

Origin

Naturally produced in humans, one of the principal substrates for the biosynthesis of macromolecules that comprise articular cartilage. For food supplements it is produced from marine exoskeletons or synthetically. Multiple salts of glucosamine are available, including glucosamine sulphate, glucosamine hydrochloride, and Nacetyl glucosamine.

Main constituents

An amino-monosaccharide.

Presumed pharmacologic action

Anti-inflammatory, increased mucopolysaccharide and collagen production in fibro-blasts in vitro, inhibition of enzymes which break down cartilage (e.g. elastase), similar actions to chondroitin (📖 see p. 142).

Commonly used dosage

500mg of glucosamine sulphate 3 times daily, observed safe level of intake is 2000mg/day.

Clinical bottom line

Benefits

😃 *Likely to be beneficial*

- Osteoarthritis: overall results for pain, function and restoration of cartilage are conflicting but there are indications that certain subgroups might respond better.

😕 *Unknown effectiveness*

- Haemostasis: poly-N-acetyl glucosamine patches at arterial puncture site in cardiac catherization, not enough data available.
- Rheumatoid arthritis: might improve symptoms but not enough data available.
- Temporomandibular joint disorders: not enough data available.

Risks

- *Contraindications:* pregnancy and lactation.
- *Precautions/warnings:* avoid use in children under the age of 2 years, in patients with asthma, or shell fish allergies. Although no significant effects on glycaemic control have been found, it is advisable to monitor those patients closely. Observed safe level of intake is 2000mg/day.
- *Adverse effects:* mild gastrointestinal complaints including nausea, heartburn, diarrhoea, and constipation, drowsiness, dyspepsia, headache, rash.
- *Interactions:* none known.

Conclusions

- Glucosamine is likely to be effective in osteoarthritis
- Generally associated with only mild gastrointestinal complaints but should be used cautiously in certain patient populations
- The risk–benefit balance of glucosamine for osteoarthritis is likely to be positive if certain patient groups such as diabetics are monitored closely

Further reading

Distler J, Anguelouch A. Evidence-based practice: review of clinical evidence on the efficacy of glucosamine and chondroitin in the treatment of osteoarthritis. *J Am Acad Nurse Pract* 2006; **18**:487–93.

Grape (*Vitis vinifera*)

Profile
Origin
Fruits, skin, seeds, and leaves of grapes have been used medicinally since the Greek empire.

Main constituents
Flavonoids, fruit acids, polyphenols (oligomeric proanthocyanidins, procyanidins), tannins, tocopherols.

Presumed pharmacologic action
Antioxidant, antimutagenic, anti-inflammatory, astringent, laxative, vasorelaxant.

Commonly used dosage
- *Grape seed extract:* 100–300mg of extract daily have been used.
- *Red vine leaf extract:* 360–720mg of daily.

Clinical bottom line
Benefits

:☺: *Beneficial*
- Cardiovascular risk: moderate wine consumption, dietary flavonol intake through red wine, red grape juice, or grape skin and seeds have cardioprotective effects.

☺ *Unknown effectiveness*
- Chronic venous insufficiency: leaf of red vine extract effective in mild symptoms and signs yet not enough data available.
- Diarrhoea: in children, white grape juice, not enough data available.
- Energy intake: some reductions noted with both red wine and grape juice but not enough data available.
- Hypercholesterolaemia: data conflicting.

☒ *Likely to be ineffective or harmful*
- Agitation in severely demented patients: aromatherapy oil of grape seed, lavender and thyme not shown to be effective.
- Radiation-induced breast induration: ineffective.
- Seasonal allergic rhinitis: no evidence of effectiveness.

Risks
- *Contraindications:* pregnancy and lactation, allergies to grapes.
- *Precautions/warnings:* might cause diarrhoea if consumed in excessive doses, alcohol content of red wine needs to be considered.
- *Adverse effects:* dry itchy scalp, headache, dizziness, and nausea with grape seed.
- *Interactions:* theoretically increases the risk of bleeding when used with anticoagulants or antiplatelet drugs. A significant interaction between grape seed and vitamin C for effects on blood pressure has been reported.

Conclusions

- Evidence exists for cardioprotective effects
- Only few risks reported although alcohol content of wine needs to be considered
- Risk–benefit balance for cardiovascular risk is positive when consumed in recommended doses

Further reading

Kar P, Laight D, Shaw KM, Cummings MH. Flavonoid-rich grapeseed extracts: a new approach in high cardiovascular risk patients? *Int J Clin Pract* 2006; **60**:1484–92.

Green tea (*Camellia sinensis*)

Profile

Origin

Black, oolong and green tea are made from the same plant and differ according to the curing method of the leaves which are used for medicinal purposes.

Main constituents

Caffeine, epigallocatechin, epigallocatechin-3-gallate

Presumed pharmacologic action

Antibacterial, antimutagenic, anticarcinogenic, antioxidant, central nervous system stimulant, anti-inflammatory.

Commonly used dosage

6–10 cups of tea or equivalent.

Clinical bottom line

Benefits

☺ *Beneficial*

- Cancer, prevention: based mostly on epidemiological data.
- Cardiovascular diseases: prevention, based mostly on epidemiological data.

☺ *Unknown effectiveness*

- AIDS: adjuvant treatment, not enough data available.
- Gingivitis: reduces inflammation but not enough data available.
- Hypercholesterolaemia: reductions of total and LDL cholesterol reported but not enough data available.
- Obesity: weight control, data contradictory.
- Papilloma virus infection: not enough data available.

Table 14.16 Systematic up-to-date review where green tea has been found to be beneficial

Condition	Source	No. of trials/ patients	Original conclusion
Breast cancer prevention	*Carcinogenesis* 2006; **27**:1310–5	N=13 (epidemiological studies)	Meta-analysis indicates a lower risk of breast cancer

Risks

- *Contraindications:* pregnancy and lactation (large doses).
- *Precautions/warnings:* none known.
- *Adverse effects:* insomnia, gastrointestinal symptoms.
- *Interactions:* none known.

Conclusions

- Can be useful in the prevention of cancer and cardiovascular conditions
- Good safety record
- For the above two indications the risk–benefit balance is positive
- Green tea is not an alternative to conventional preventive strategy but should be considered as an integral part of it

Further reading

Beltz LA, Bayer DK, Moss AL, Simet IM. Mechanisms of cancer prevention by green and black tea polyphenols. *Anticancer Agents Med Chem* 2006; **6**:389–406.

Fraser ML, Mok GS, Lee AH. Green tea and stroke prevention: emerging evidence. *Complement Ther Med* 2007; **15**:46–53.

Green-lipped mussel (*Perna canaliculus*)

Profile
Origin
Tissue from the New Zealand *Perna canaliculus* is freeze dried and used as a dietary supplement.

Main constituents
Omega-3 fatty acids.

Presumed pharmacologic action
Anti-inflammatory.

Commonly used dosage
900–1200mg mussel extract per day.

Clinical bottom line
Benefits

☹ *Unknown effectiveness*
- Osteoarthritis, pain, function: data conflicting.
- Rheumatoid arthritis, pain, function: data conflicting.

Risks
- *Contraindications:* pregnancy and lactation, hypercoagulability.
- *Precautions/warnings:* may act as a COX2 inhibitor.
- *Adverse effects:* none known.
- *Interactions:* anticoagulants.

Conclusions

- Effectiveness is not clearly demonstrated
- Only minor risks on record
- The risk–benefit balance fails to be positive for any condition

Further reading
Cobb CS, Ernst E. Systematic review of a marine nutriceutical supplement in clinical trials for arthritis: the effectiveness of the New Zealand green-lipped mussel *Perna canaliculus*. *Clin Rheumatol* 2006; **25**: 275–84.

Guar gum

Profile

Origin

Guar gum is derived from the Indian cluster bean (*Cyamopsis tetra-gonolobas*). It is a plant-based dietary fibre that has been advocated for type 2 diabetes and hypercholesterolaemia. It is used widely by the food and other industries as thickening agent in, for instance, diary products (EU food additive code E412).

Main constituents

Galactomannan.

Presumed pharmacologic action

Laxative, antihyperlipidaemic, antihyperglycaemic.

Commonly used dosage

9–15g daily orally.

Clinical bottom line

Benefits

:☻: *Beneficial*

- Hypercholesterolaemia: lowers total and LDL cholesterol.

☻ *Likely to be beneficial*

- Irritable bowel syndrome: seems to improve gastrointestinal symptoms.

☹ *Unknown effectiveness*

- Constipation: may increase faecal output in elderly hospitalized patients.
- Diabetes type 1 and 2: may improve fasting blood glucose yet not enough data available.
- Diarrhoea: seems to reduce duration of diarrhoea in children and diarrhoeal episodes in patients on enteral nutrition but not enough data available.
- Duodenal ulcer: may improve symptoms yet not enough data available.
- Hypotension: postprandial hypotension may be attenuated yet not enough data available.

☹ *Unlikely to be beneficial*

- Cholestasis: unlikely to have effects on pruritus, bile salts, fetal, or neonatal outcomes in pregnant women.

☒ *Likely to be ineffective or harmful*

- Body weight reduction: ineffective for reducing body weight or feeling of hunger.

Risks

- *Contraindications:* pregnancy and lactation.
- *Precautions/warnings:* should be taken with sufficient amounts of fluid.

- *Adverse effects:* allergic reactions, flatulence, diarrhoea, abdominal pain, cramps.
- *Interactions:* possible potentiation of the effects of insulin, decreased absorption of oral contraceptives.

Conclusions

- Guar gum lowers total and LDL cholesterol in hypercholesterolaemic patients: it is likely to be effective in irritable bowel syndrome
- Risk of adverse events and drug interactions exist
- The risk–benefit balance seems positive for hypercholesterolaemia and likely to be positive for irritable bowel syndrome if adverse events and interactions are avoided
- Guar gum seems a beneficial adjunct to diet and conventional options for treating hypercholesterolaemia

Further reading

Giannini EG, Mansi C, Dulbecco P, Savarino V. Role of partially hydrolyzed guar gum in the treatment of irritable bowel syndrome. *Nutrition* 2006; **22**:334–42.

Hawthorn (*Crataegus* spp)

Profile

Origin
Crataegus species are native to the temperate regions of North America, Asia and Europe. *Crataegus* species found in hawthorn preparations include mainly *C. laevigata* and *C. monogyna*.

Main constituents
Catechin, epicatechin, flavonoids (quercetin, hyperoside, vitexin, rutin), procyanidins.

Presumed pharmacologic action
Dilation of coronary arteries, positive inotropic, decrease of atrioventricular conduction time and increase of refractory period, cardioprotective, antiarrhythmic, hypotensive, beta-blocking and ACE-inhibiting activity, antioxidant, central nervous system depressant. The mechanism of action is similar to digitalis.

Commonly used dosage
900mg standardized (2.2% flavonoids or 18.75% oligomeric procyanidines) extract daily.

Clinical bottom line

Benefits

:☺: *Beneficial*
- Chronic heart failure: beneficial effects for maximal workload and the pressure heart rate product in mild-to-moderate conditions.

☺ *Unknown effectiveness*
- Anxiety, mild-to-moderate: some positive yet not enough data exist.
- Hypertension: may have hypotensive effects yet not enough data available.
- Hypotension, orthostatic: tested in a combination preparation with camphor showing some positive evidence but more data required.

Table 4.17 Systematic up-to-date review where hawthorn has been found to be beneficial

Condition	Source	No. of trials/ patients	Original conclusion
Chronic heart failure	*Cochrane Database Syst Rev* (in press)	N=14/n=1110	Hawthorn extract has significant benefits, compared with placebo, as an adjunctive treatment for patients with chronic heart failure. Reported adverse events were infrequent, mild, and transient

Risks

- *Contraindications:* pregnancy and lactation, allergy to plants from the *Rosaceae* family.
- *Precautions/warnings:* sedation, hypotension, or arrhythmias with high doses; hawthorn should only be used under medical supervision.
- *Adverse effects:* nausea, dizziness, vertigo, fatigue, sweating, palpitations, tachycardia, gastrointestinal complaints.
- *Interactions:* additive effects with antihypertensive drugs, nitrates, cardiac glycosides and central nervous system depressants.

Conclusions

- There is benefit over placebo from hawthorn extract as an adjunctive treatment for chronic heart failure
- Its safety profile is encouraging: only mild and infrequent adverse events have been reported
- For chronic heart failure the risk–benefit balance is positive, however, due to the nature of the condition, close medical supervision is essential

Further reading

Daniele C, Mazzanti G, Pittler MH, Ernst E. Adverse-event profile of *Crataegus* spp.: a systematic review. *Drug Saf* 2006; **29**:523–35.

Hop (*Humulus lupulus*)

Profile
Origin
A climbing perennial herb belonging to the *Cannabaceae* family, found in marshy areas throughout Asia, the United States, and Europe. As well as being crucial to the brewing industry, hop has a long history of use as a sedative. Female flowering parts (strobiles) are used for medicinal purposes.

Main constituents
Chalcones, flavonoids, oleo-resin, tannins, volatile oils.

Presumed pharmacologic action
Sedative, antimicrobial.

Commonly used dosage
- *Dried extract:* 0.5–1g 3 times daily
- *Liquid extract:* 0.5–1mL (1:1 in 45% alcohol) 3 times daily
- 84mg hops extract combined with 374mg valerian taken once before bedtime.

Clinical bottom line
Benefits

😕 *Unknown effectiveness*
- Menopausal discomfort: 8-prenylnaringenin enriched extract, not enough data available.
- Sleep: possible hypnotic effects suggested for hops/valerian combination products yet the role of hops on its own is unclear.

Risks
- *Contraindications:* pregnancy and lactation, depression.
- *Precautions/warnings:* may have oestrogenic agonist or antagonist properties, with unknown effects on hormone sensitive conditions; disruption to menstrual cycle is considered possible. Might potentially increase blood sugar levels in diabetic patients.
- *Adverse effects:* allergic dermatitis, respiratory allergy and anaphylaxis have been reported following inhalation or external contact with the herb or oil.
- *Interactions:* theoretical interactions exist for central nervous system depressants, antipsychotics, hormonal agents and any drugs metabolized by the cytochrome P-450 system.

Conclusions

- There is insufficient clinical data to suggest that hop has any specific therapeutic effect
- Conclusive safety information is also lacking, but some risks have been identified
- The risk–benefit balance is not positive for any condition

Further reading

Chadwick LR, Pauli GF, Farnsworth NR. The pharmacognosy of *Humulus lupulus* L. (hops) with an emphasis on estrogenic properties. *Phytomedicine* 2006; **13**:119–31.

Horse chestnut (*Aesculus hippocastanum*)

Profile

Origin

The horse chestnut tree is native to south-east Europe. Today it is widely distributed all over the world. The seeds are used for medicinal purposes.

Main constituents

Fatty acids, flavonoids, quinones, saponins, sterols, tannins, and triterpene. The principal active component of horse chestnut seed extract is escin.

Presumed pharmacologic action

Antiexudative, anti-inflammatory and immunomodulatory activity.

Commonly used dosage

- *Internal use:* extract standardized to 100–150mg escin daily in divided doses.
- *External use:* apply several times daily.

Clinical bottom line

Benefits

:☻: *Beneficial*

- Chronic venous insufficiency: leg oedema, mild-to-moderate leg pain, tenseness and fatigue.

Table 4.18 Systematic up-to-date review where horse chestnut has been found to be beneficial

Condition	Source	No. of trials/patients	Original conclusion
Chronic venous insufficiency	*Cochrane Database Syst Rev* 2006; **1**:CD003230	N=17/n=1581	Horse chestnut seed extract appears to be effective and safe as a symptomatic, short-term treatment for CVI

Risks

- *Contraindications:* pregnancy and lactation, bleeding disorders, allergy to any of its constituents.
- *Precautions/warnings:* open wounds, weeping eczema (external use), intravenous administration.
- *Adverse effects:* pruritus, nausea, gastrointestinal complaints, bleeding, dizziness, headache, nephropathy, allergic reactions.
- *Interactions:* increased effects of aspirin and other anticoagulants, anti-hyperglycaemics.

Conclusions

- Horse chestnut seed extract is effective for chronic venous insufficiency
- Only mild and infrequent adverse events have been reported
- The risk–benefit balance is positive for chronic venous insufficiency

Indian frankincense (*Boswellia serrata*)

Profile

Origin
A tree found in India, North Africa, and the Middle East. Its bark exudes a resinous gum which is used medicinally. Traditionally used in Ayurvedic medicine.

Main constituents
Boswellic acid, alpha-boswellic acid.

Presumed pharmacologic action
Analgesic, anti-inflammatory, inhibits the enzyme 5-lipoxygenase and glucosaminoglycan synthesis.

Commonly used dosage
Between 300–1200mg, 3 times daily.

Clinical bottom line

Benefits

😑 *Unknown effectiveness*
- Asthma: encouraging results for chronic therapy but not enough data available.
- Colitis: microscopic and collagenous, not enough data available.
- Colitis, ulcerative: only limited evidence available
- Crohn's disease: combination products used, not enough data available.
- Osteoarthritis: encouraging results for pain reduction but methodological limitation, not enough data available.

😟 *Unlikely to be beneficial*
- Rheumatoid arthritis: no beneficial effects on pain and swelling reported.

Risks
- *Contraindications:* pregnancy and lactation, may be an emmenagogue and induce abortion.
- *Precautions/warnings:* use cautiously in patients taking lipid-soluble medication, patients with gastritis or gastro-oesophageal reflux disease.
- *Adverse effects:* nausea, acid reflux, mild gastrointestinal upset.
- *Interactions:* may potentiate the action of leukotriene inhibitors, lipid-lowering agents, antineoplastic agents.

Conclusions

- There is insufficient evidence of effectiveness available for any condition
- Risks are usually of a mild nature, mainly gastrointestinal complaints
- The risk–benefit balance fails to be positive for any condition

Further reading

Basch E, Boon H, Davies-Heerema T et al. Boswellia: an evidence-based systematic review by the Natural Standard Research Collaboration. *J Herb Pharmacother 2004*; **4**:63–83.

Kava (*Piper methysticum*)

Profile

Origin

Kava is native to the South Pacific: it is prepared from the rhizome of *Piper methysticum*.

Main constituents

Dihydrokavain, dihydromethysticin, kavain, methysticin, yangonin.

Presumed pharmacologic action

Anxiolytic, sedative, anaesthetic, muscle relaxant. Kavapyrones are the pharmacologically active components, and act on the central nervous system. They are thought to mediate effects on gamma-aminobutyric acid receptors.

Commonly used dosage

300mg of standardized extract (210mg kavapyrones) daily in divided doses.

Clinical bottom line

Benefits

🆗 *Trade off between benefits and harms:*

- Anxiety: effective for symptom control but serious safety issues including liver damage exist.

😐 *Unknown effectiveness*

- Cognitive function: may enhance memory and increase positive affectivity but not enough data available.
- Insomnia: may improve quality of sleep but data limited.
- Menopause: may improve symptoms but not enough data available.

Table 4.19 Systematic up-to-date reviews where kava has been found to be effective

Condition	Source	No. of trials/ patients	Original conclusion
Anxiety	*Cochrane Database Syst Rev* 2003; **1**:CD003383	N=12/n=700	Compared with placebo, kava extract is an effective symptomatic treatment for anxiety although, at present, the size of the effect seems to be small

Risks

- *Contraindications:* pregnancy and lactation, endogenous depression, allergy, liver conditions, Parkinson's disease.
- *Precautions/warnings:* avoid long-term use. The extract can cause visual disturbances and may affect reaction time. Care must be taken when driving or operating machinery.

- *Adverse effects:* stomach complaints, tremor, headache, drowsiness, restlessness, dyskinesia, mydriasis, allergic skin reactions, kava dermopathy, dermatomyositis, liver damage.
- *Interactions:* potentiation of drugs acting on the central nervous system such as alcohol, benzodiazepines, barbiturates and anaesthetics: may potentiate the effects of hepatotoxic agents: may reduce the effects of levodopa.

Conclusions

- Best evidence suggests that kava is effective for treating anxiety
- Serious safety issues exist particularly regarding liver damage
- The risk–benefit balance is not clearly positive for treating anxiety
  It should only be taken short-term and under close medical observation

Further reading

Ulbricht C, Basch E, Boon H et al. Safety review of kava (Piper methysticum) by the Natural Standard Research Collaboration. *Expert Opin Drug Saf* 2005; **4**:779–94.

Bladderwrack (*Fucus vesiculosus*)

Profile

Origin
A brown seaweed of the *Fucaceae* family which grows in the Atlantic and Pacific oceans, the North and Baltic seas.

Main constituents
Iodine, other ingredients are likely but have not yet been identified.

Presumed pharmacologic action
Stimulation of the thyroid, therefore used for weight reduction: hypoglycaemic, anticoagulant, antimicrobial, laxative, antioxidant.

Commonly used dosage
Thyroid disease, weight loss: 200–600mg extract/day.

Clinical bottom line

Benefits

😐 *Unknown effectiveness*
- Cervical ripening: data contradictory.
- Thyroid function: might increase thyroid-stimulating hormone but not enough data available.

Risks
- *Contraindications:* thyroid disease, diabetes, pregnancy and lactation.
- *Precautions/warnings:* regular intake can cause thyroid disease, heavy metal contamination possible.
- *Adverse effects:* increases thyroid-stimulating hormone, acne, diarrhoea.
- *Interactions:* anticoagulants, antidiabetics, medication for thyroid disease, central nervous system stimulants, lithium.

Conclusions

- There is no evidence available that bladderwrack is effective for any indication
- Considerable risks have been documented
- The risk–benefit balance is negative

Kombucha

Profile

Origin

An aggregate of yeast and bacteria in a semi-permeable membrane, used to make a 'tea' which is recommended for general wellbeing and a range of medical conditions. Pronounced /com-boo-cha/.

Main constituents

Acetic acid, alcohol, B vitamins, chondroitin-sulphate, glucoronic acid, hyalronic acid, heparin, lactic acid, mukoitin sulphate, usnic acid, sugar.

Presumed pharmacologic action

Antioxidant, immunomodulation, hepatoprotection.

Commonly used dosage

Tea is consumed several times per day.

Clinical bottom line

Benefits

☹ *Unknown effectiveness*
- There is no trial data available for any indication.

Risks

- *Contraindications:* pregnancy and lactation.
- *Precautions/warnings:* tea can contain alcohol and toxic chemicals.
- *Adverse effects:* liver damage, infection (e.g. anthrax), allergic reactions.
- *Interactions:* none known.

Conclusions

- No benefit has been documented for any conditions
- Serious adverse effects are on record
- The risk–benefit balance is clearly negative
- The use of kombucha as a medicine should be discouraged

Laetrile

Profile

Origin

Laetrile is a semi-synthetic derivate of amygdalin which is a glycoside from apricot kernels. Also sometimes named vitamin B_{17}.

Main constituent

Amygdalin.

Presumed pharmacologic action

Anti-neoplastic.

Commonly used dosage

3–12g per day.

Clinical bottom line

Benefits

⚔ *Likely to be ineffective or harmful*
- Cancer: there is no evidence of effectiveness and potential for considerable harm.

Risks

- *Contraindications:* laetrile is toxic.
- *Precautions/warnings:* laetrile is toxic.
- *Adverse effects:* cyanide poisoning.
- *Interactions:* not known.

Conclusions

- No reliable evidence for effectiveness for any type of cancer
- There is considerable potential for harm, e.g. cyanide poisoning
- The risk–benefit balance is negative

Further reading

Milazzo S, Ernst E, Lejeune S, Schmidt K. Laetrile treatment for cancer. *Cochrane Database Syst Rev* 2006; **2**:CD005476.

Lavender (*Lavandula angustifolia*)

Profile

Origin

Native to the Mediterranean, widely cultivated in domestic gardens and for use in perfumes and toiletries. Its name is derived from the Latin *lavare* (to wash). Flowering tops are used for medicinal purposes.

Main constituents

Camphor, cineole, flavonoids, hydroxycoumarins, limonene, perillyl alcohol, tannins, triterpens, volatile oil (linalyl acetate, linalool).

Presumed pharmacologic action

Astringent, sedative, anticonvulsant, antioxidant, lipid lowering.

Commonly used dosage

- *Tea:* 1–2 teaspoons of dried flowers in 150mL of hot water.
- *Inhalation:* 2–4 drops of oil in 2–3 cups of boiling water.

Clinical bottom line

Benefits

🙂 *Unknown effectiveness*
- Insomnia: not enough data available.
- Mood: only few and methodologically limited data available for mood including depression, stress, agitated behaviour.
- Work performance: might improve concentration levels but only few data available.

😖 *Unlikely to be beneficial*
- Pain: no effect on various pain syndromes including experimentally induced pain, cancer pain, postnatal perineal discomfort.
- Recovery from exercise: no effect of lavender oil aromatherapy.

Risks

- *Contraindications:* pregnancy and lactation.
- *Precautions/warnings:* the essential oil should be regarded as potentially poisonous if taken internally.
- *Adverse effects:* nausea, vomiting, headache and chills have been reported following inhalation or absorption through the skin. Contact allergy and phototoxicity are also possible.
- *Interactions:* could theoretically potentiate effects of central nervous system depressants.

Conclusions

- Some trials suggest that lavender has relaxing effects yet the evidence from clinical trials does not show that it has specific therapeutic effects for any condition
- In recommended doses generally considered well-tolerated with some adverse events
- The risk–benefit balance is not positive

Further reading

Basch E, Foppa I, Liebowitz R et al. Lavender (*Lavandula angustifolia* Miller). *J Herb Pharmacother* 2004; **4**:63–78.

Lemon balm (*Melissa officinalis*)

Profile

Origin
A perennial plant from the Mediterranean and West Asia; leaves (which smell of lemon) are used for medicinal purposes.

Main constituents
Monoterpinoid aldehydes (e.g. *Citronella* L), flavonoids, monoterpene, glycosides.

Presumed pharmacologic action
Sedative, antimicrobial, spasmolytic, inhibition of lipid peroxidation, anti-inflammatory.

Commonly used dosage
- Topical: 1% cream, 3 times daily.
- 1.5–4.5g of dried leaf or equivalent.

Clinical bottom line

Benefits

😐 *Unknown effectiveness*
- Agitation in dementia (essential oil used for aromatherapy): not enough data available.
- Alzheimer's disease: not enough data available.
- Anxiety: not enough data available.
- Herpes labialis (topical application): data suggest that lesions heal quicker and symptoms are less severe but not enough data available.
- Stress: not enough data available.

Risks
- *Contraindications:* pregnancy (oral) and lactation.
- *Precautions/warnings:* none.
- *Adverse effects:* allergic reactions.
- *Interactions:* can enhance effects of sedatives.

Conclusions

- The effectiveness of lemon balm has not been convincingly demonstrated for any indications
- No serious risks are on record
- The risk–benefit balance fails to be positive

Further reading

Ulbricht C, Brendler T, Gruenwald J *et al.* Lemon balm (*Melissa officinalis* L.): an evidence-based systematic review by the Natural Standard Research Collaboration. *J Herb Pharmacother* 2005; **5**:71–114.

Liquorice (*Glycyrrhiza glabra*)

Profile

Origin
Liquorice is extracted from the root of *Glycyrrhiza glabra*, which is a legume and related to beans and peas. It is a herbaceous perennial and native to southern Europe and parts of Asia. Liquorice flavour is found in a wide variety of sweets.

Main constituents
Glycyrrhizin.

Presumed pharmacologic action
Laxative, expectorant, hypertensive (11β-hydroxysteroid dehydrogenase inhibition and cortisol increase).

Commonly used dosage
1–3g of extract daily.

Clinical bottom line

Benefits

😃 *Likely to be beneficial*
- Functional dyspepsia: a combination preparation (STW5) seems to improve gastrointestinal symptoms.

😐 *Unknown effectiveness*
- Arthritis, rheumatoid: not enough data available.
- Atopic dermatitis: a topical gel may reduce symptoms but not enough data available.
- Hepatitis C, chronic: may improve virological and biochemical markers but data inconclusive.
- Mediterranean fever: a combination preparation (Guard®) may improve duration, severity and frequency of attacks but not enough data available.
- Thrombocytopenic purpura: not enough data available.

Risks
- *Contraindications:* hypertension, chronic heart failure, kidney and liver disease, oedema, pregnancy and lactation.
- *Precautions/warnings:* blood pressure increase, hypokalaemia.
- *Adverse effects:* headache, nausea, gastrointestinal complaints, allergic reactions, arrhythmia, fluid retention.
- *Interactions:* may increase digoxin toxicity, reduce effects of diuretic or anti-hypertensive drugs.

Conclusions

- Best evidence suggests that the combination preparation STW5 is likely to be beneficial for functional dyspepsia, the role of liquorice on its own is, however, unclear
- Adverse effects have been reported and may be serious
- The risk–benefit ratio is not convincingly positive for any condition

Marigold (*Calendula officinalis*)

Profile

Origin
Also known as marigold, this annual flower of the daisy family is native to Asia and Southern Europe. Flowers are used for medicinal purposes. Calendula is mostly used topically.

Main constituents
Triterpenoids and flavonoids.

Presumed pharmacologic action
Anti-inflammatory, immuno-stimulating, anti-microbial, sedation, anti-hypertensive, wound healing.

Commonly used dosage
2–5% ointments applied 3 times per day.

Clinical bottom line

Benefits

☻ *Unknown effectiveness*
- Contact dermatitis: not enough data available.
- Radiation dermatitis: not enough data available.
- Venous leg ulcers: not enough data available.

Risks
- *Contraindications:* none.
- *Precautions/warnings:* pregnancy and lactation.
- *Adverse effects:* allergic reactions.
- *Interactions:* none known with topical use.

Conclusions

- Topical use of marigold is not supported by sound evidence for any condition. For oral use, no reliable data exist
- Only minor and rare risks are known
- The risk–benefit balance fails to be positive for any condition

Further reading

Basch E, Bent S, Foppa *et al.* Marigold (*Calendula officinalis* L.): an evidence-based systematic review by the Natural Standard Research Collaboration. *J Herb Pharmacother* 2006; **6**:135–59.

Melatonin

Profile

Origin

Melatonin is a neurohormone synthesized from tryptophan. Release is stimulated by darkness and suppressed by light. It is involved in the regulation of bodily rhythms such as temperature and sleep. Melatonin is produced endogenously but also available commercially as synthetic preparations.

Presumed pharmacologic action

Synchronizing hormone secretion, sedative, antioxidative, immune stimulating, antiproliferative, anti-inflammatory, hypotensive.

Commonly used dosage

- *Insomnia:* 0.3–10mg (0.3–1mg initially) 1 to 2 hours before bedtime.
- *Jet lag:* 5mg 22–2400 hrs local time on arrival for 4 days.

Clinical bottom line

Benefits

:☺: *Beneficial*

- Insomnia: improves sleep quality.
- Jet lag: taken close to bedtime at the destination decreases jet-lag when crossing five or more time zones.

☺ *Likely to be beneficial*

- Irritable bowel syndrome: may improve abdominal pain and overall symptom scores.

☻ *Unknown effectiveness*

- Adjunct to pre-operative medication: not enough data available.
- Alopecia, diffuse or androgenic: not enough data available.
- Benign prostatic hyperplasia: not enough data available.
- Cancer, treatment: might prolong survival time yet more methodologically rigorous data required.
- Cluster headache: not enough data available.
- Dementia, motor restlessness: not enough data available.
- Diabetes, type 2: may improve glycaemic control but not enough data available.
- Epilepsy: not enough data available.
- Gastroesophageal reflux: may relieve symptoms yet not enough data available.
- Hypertension: small reduction of nocturnal systolic and diastolic blood pressures but not enough data available.
- Tardive dyskinesia: not enough data available.
- Whiplash syndrome: not enough data available.

✗ *Likely to be ineffective or harmful*

- Anxiety: no effects in elderly patients undergoing surgery.
- Chronic fatigue syndrome: likely to be ineffective.
- Menopause: no relief of symptoms.

- Sedation: unlikely to improve sedation with standard oral regimen.
- Tinnitus: likely to be ineffective.

Risks

- *Contraindications:* pregnancy and lactation, prepubertal children, autoimmune disease, hepatic insufficiency, cerebrovascular or neurologic disorders, patients taking immunosuppressants or corticosteroids.
- *Precautions/warnings:* impairment of psychomotor vigilance. Driving or operating machinery should be avoided for 4–5 hours following melatonin administration. Melatonin may be pro-atherosclerotic.
- *Adverse effects:* abdominal cramps, fatigue, dizziness, headache, irritability. Hangover effects are unlikely, due to the short half-life.
- *Interactions:* may potentiate the effects of benzodiazepines and antihypertensive drugs. May reduce the effects of warfarin and antihyperglycaemic drugs.

Conclusions

- Effective in preventing or reducing jet-lag and in improving sleep quality in patients with insomnia. Likely to be beneficial in irritable bowel syndrome
- The short-term safety profile seems to be favourable
- The risk–benefit balance is positive for jet lag and for improving sleep quality and likely to be positive for irritable bowel syndrome

Further reading

Ruddick JP, Evans AK, Nutt DJ *et al.* Tryptophan metabolism in the central nervous system: medical implications. *Expert Rev Mol Med* 2006; **8**:1–27.

Milk thistle (*Silybum marianum*)

Profile

Origin
Milk thistle belongs to the *Compositae* (*Asteraceae*) family and is native to the Mediterranean. Seeds are used for medicinal purposes.

Main constituents
Silymarin which is composed of the flavoligans silybin, silychristin, and silydianin.

Presumed pharmacologic action
Alters the membrane structure of liver cells so that toxins are hindered from entering hepatocytes, increases their regenerative capacity, competes with binding sites for liver toxins; antioxidant, free radical scavenger and possibly cholesterol-lowering agent.

Commonly used dosage
160–480mg of standardized extract (70–80% silymarin) 3 times daily. Silymarin is not soluble in water, therefore ineffective when taken as tea.

Clinical bottom line

Benefits

😃 *Likely to be beneficial*
- Hepatitis, viral: likely to decrease serum transaminases.

😐 *Unknown effectiveness*
- Diabetes: beneficial effects on glycaemic profile but not enough data available.

🙁 *Likely to be ineffective or harmful*
- Liver disease (alcoholic liver and/or viral hepatitis B or C): no significant effect on all-cause mortality, complications of liver disease or liver histology.

Risks
- *Contraindications:* pregnancy and lactation.
- *Precautions/warnings:* intake for an extended duration. Caution in patients with diabetes or taking hypoglycaemic agents.
- *Adverse effects:* mild gastrointestinal complaints, diarrhoea, pruritus, headache, rare cases of anaphylaxis.
- *Interactions:* theoretically, improvement of liver function could increase metabolism of some medications metabolized in the liver; preliminary evidence that milk thistle might inhibit cytochrome P450.

Conclusions

- Not demonstrably effective in any condition but likely to be beneficial in viral hepatitis
- No serious risks are on record but interactions need to be considered
- The risk–benefit balance fails to be convincingly positive for any condition but it might be positive for viral hepatitis

Further reading

Rambaldi A, Jacobs BP, Iaquinto G, Gluud C. Milk thistle for alcoholic and/or hepatitis B or C virus liver diseases. *Cochrane Database Syst Rev* 2005; **2**:CD003620.

Mistletoe (*Viscum album*)

Profile

Origin
Leaves, branches and berries of *Viscum album* are used. Depending on which host tree the parasitic mistletoe grows on, its actions are said to be slightly different.

Main constituents
Mistletoe lectins.

Presumed pharmacologic action
Cytotoxic, stimulation of immune defence.

Commonly used dosage
Various dosing regimen are used and many depend on the condition and nature of extract.

Clinical bottom line

Benefits

☻ *Unknown effectiveness*
- Cancer: reduction of tumour burden, improvement of quality of life, tolerability of cancer treatments, trial data contradictory and methodologically limited.
- Common cold: symptom control, not enough data available.
- Hepatitis C, symptom control: not enough data available.

Risks
- *Contraindications:* pregnancy and lactation.
- *Precautions/warnings:* do not use as an alternative to conventional therapy.
- *Adverse effects:* bradycardia, dehydration, delirium, hepatitis, fever, leukocytosis, seizures, vomiting.
- *Interactions:* antihypertensives, cardiac and CNS depressants.

Conclusions

- Effectiveness has not been demonstrated
- Considerable risks have been noted
- The risk–benefit balance fails to be positive
- Mistletoe does not have proven effectiveness for any of the conditions it is promoted for; many, in particular cancer, can be treated more effectively by conventional healthcare

Further reading

Kienle GS, Kiene H. Complementary cancer therapy: a systematic review of prospective clinical trials on anthroposophic mistletoe extracts. *Eur J Med Res 2007*; **12**:103–19.

Nettle (*Urtica dioica*)

Profile

Origin

A perennial herb, which grows throughout much of the temperate zones of both hemispheres. It is considered a weed and causes a characteristic itching rash upon contact with the skin. Leaves and roots are used for medicinal purposes.

Main constituents

- *Leaf*: minerals, flavonoids, sterols, tannins, vitamins.
- *Root*: coumarin, fatty acids, lectins, lignans, polysaccharides, sterols, tannins, terpenes.

Presumed pharmacologic action

Diuretic, analgesic, antihypertensive, immunostimulatory and anti-inflammatory.

Commonly used dosage

- *Leaf*: 0.6–2.1g of dry extract daily in divided doses.
- *Root*: 0.7–1.3g of dry extract daily in divided doses.

Clinical bottom line

Benefits

😊 *Likely to be beneficial*

- Benign prostatic hyperplasia: seems to improve lower urinary tract symptoms.

😐 *Unknown effectiveness*

- Osteoarthritis: some beneficial effects are reported but not enough data available.
- Seasonal allergic rhinitis: may improve symptoms but data are scarce and have methodological limitations.

Risks

- *Contraindications*: pregnancy and lactation.
- *Precautions/warnings*: children under the age of 2 years.
- *Adverse effects*: gastrointestinal complaints, diarrhoea, allergic reactions, urticaria, pruritus, oedema, decreased urine volume.
- *Interactions*: may potentiate the effects of diuretic, antihypertensive, antihyperglycaemic, central nervous system depressant agents: might decrease the effects of anticoagulant drugs.

Conclusions

- Best evidence suggests that nettle root extract is likely beneficial for benign prostatic hyperplasia
- There are only mild and infrequent adverse events
- The risk–benefit balance for benign prostatic hyperplasia is likely to be positive

Passion flower (*Passiflora incarnata*)

Profile

Origin

A perennial vine native to the Americas. Its flowered fringe is thought to represent the crown of thorns and its five anthers represent the five stigmata: the Latin name means suffering *(passio)* and incarnate *(incarnata)*. Aerial parts, particularly leaves are used for medicinal purposes. Most commonly used in combination with other herbs.

Main constituents

Alkaloids, coumarin derivatives, fatty acids, flavonoids, maltol.

Presumed pharmacologic action

Sedative, hypnotic, anxiolytic, antispasmolytic.

Commonly used dosage

- *Aerial parts:* 0.25–2g of the dried above ground parts, 3 times daily.
- *Liquid extract:* 0.5–1mL (1:1 in 25% alcohol) 3 times daily.
- *Tincture:* 0.5–1mL (1:8 in 45% alcohol) 3 times daily.

Clinical bottom line

Benefits

😐 *Unknown effectiveness*

- Anxiety: encouraging results for generalized anxiety disorders; herbal combination reduced anxiety in adjustment disorder but not enough data available.
- Drug dependence, opiate withdrawal symptoms: in combination with clonidine better than clonidine alone in reducing anxiety, irritability, insomnia and agitation but not enough data available.
- Dyspnoea: in combination with hawthorn improvements in the physical exercise capacity yet not enough data available.

Risks

- *Contraindications:* pregnancy and lactation.
- *Precautions/warnings:* ability to drive or operate machinery may be impaired.
- *Adverse effects:* dizziness, confusion, ataxia, nausea, vomiting, drowsiness, ventricular tachycardia, and vasculitis have been reported.
- *Interactions:* theoretically potentiation of drugs with sedative properties and anticoagulant/antiplatelet potential is possible.

Conclusions

- There is no convincing evidence for any condition
- Only few adverse events reported yet comprehensive safety data are lacking
- The risk–benefit balance is not positive for any conditions

Further reading

Miyasaka L, Atallah A, Soares B. Passiflora for anxiety disorder. *Cochrane Database Syst Rev* 2007; **1**:CD004518.

Peppermint (*Mentha x piperita*)

Profile

Origin

A perennial herb, which grows in moist regions throughout much of Europe and North America. Characterized by its smell and its square stem, which is typical for members of the mint family. A natural hybrid of water mint (*Mentha aquatica*) and spearmint (*Mentha spicata*).

Main constituents

- *Leaf:* chlorogenic and rosmarinic acids, hesperidin, luteolin, rutin, volatile oil.
- *Oil:* cineol, isomenthone, limonene, menthofuran, menthol, menthone, menthyl acetate.

Presumed pharmacologic action

Antispasmodic, antimicrobial, antiseptic, carminative, cholagogue, cooling. The principal active constituent of peppermint oil is thought to be menthol, a cyclic monoterpene with calcium channel-blocking activity.

Commonly used dosage

- *Leaf:* 3–6g as infusion daily. 0.8–1.8g of dry extract daily in divided doses.
- *Essential oil:* 0.6–1.2mL in enteric-coated capsules daily. 3–4 drops, 3 times daily in hot water internally (as inhalant). Apply as needed externally.

Clinical bottom line

Benefits

😊 *Beneficial*

- Non-ulcer dyspepsia: combination preparation of peppermint and caraway (*Carum carvi*) reduces symptoms.

😊 *Likely to be beneficial*

- Irritable bowel syndrome: may be helpful in global improvement of symptoms.
- Procedure-related gastro-intestinal spasm: seems to exert antispasmodic effects during upper endoscopy and barium meal examination.

😊 *Unknown effectiveness*

- Headache, tension-type: externally applied peppermint oil yet not enough data available.
- Nausea, postoperative: not enough data available.
- Urinary tract infection: not enough data available.

Table 4.20 Systematic up-to-date reviews where peppermint has been found to be beneficial or likely to be beneficial

Condition	Source	No. of trials/ patients	Original conclusion
Non-ulcer dyspepsia	*Aliment Pharmacol Ther* 2002; **16**:1689–99	N=9/n=1001	Some of the herbal medicinal products identified, in particular peppermint and caraway, with effects of similar or greater magnitude to conventional therapies and encouraging safety profiles, undoubtedly warrant further investigation
Irritable bowel syndrome	*Phytomedicine* 2005; **12**:601–6	N=16/n=651	Taking into account the currently available drug treatments for IBS, peppermint oil (1–2 capsules t.i.d. over 24 weeks) may be the drug of first choice in IBS patients with non-serious constipation or diarrhoea to alleviate general symptoms and to improve quality of life

Risks

- *Contraindications:* pregnancy and lactation, children under the age of 12 years, obstruction of the bile duct, cholecystitis, allergy to any constituent of peppermint.
- *Precautions/warnings:* individuals with glucose-6 phosphate dehydrogenase deficiency, gallstones, hiatal hernia.
- *Adverse effects:* allergic reactions, skin irritation, contact dermatitis, laryngeal or bronchial spasm, mouth ulceration, eye irritation, heartburn, belching, perianal burning, gastrointestinal complaints, headache, dizziness, pruritus.
- *Interactions:* might increase levels of drugs metabolized by CYP3A4.

Conclusions

- Best evidence suggests beneficial effects for non-ulcer dyspepsia; likely to be beneficial for irritable bowel syndrome and procedure-related gastrointestinal spasms
- Generally, peppermint has a good safety profile but the possibility of adverse effects exists
- The risk–benefit balance is positive for non-ulcer dyspepsia using a combination preparation and likely to be positive for irritable bowel syndrome and procedure-related gastrointestinal spasms

Further reading

Charrois TL, Hrudey J, Gardiner P, Vohra S: American Academy of Pediatrics Provisional Section on Complementary, Holistic, and Integrative Medicine. Peppermint oil. *Pediatr Rev* 2006; **27**:e49–51.

McKay DL, Blumberg JB. A review of the bioactivity and potential health benefits of peppermint tea (*Mentha piperita* L.). *Phytother Res* 2006; **20**:619–33.

Phytoestrogens

Profile

Origin
Phytoestrogens are plant-derived compounds with weak oestrogen-like activities. Certain foods such as soy-derived products are known to have high levels of phytoestrogens.

Main constituents
Coumestans, isoflavones, lignans.

Presumed pharmacologic action
Oestrogenic, antioestrogenic, proliferative, antiproliferative, antioxidative, anti-inflammatory.

Commonly used dosage
40–100mg of isoflavones daily.

Clinical bottom line

Benefits

😊 *Beneficial*
- Lipid profiles, soy: reduces total cholesterol, LDL cholesterol, triglyceride levels, increases HDL.

🙂 *Likely to be beneficial*
- Cancer, breast, soy: may be associated with a small reduction in risk.
- Cancer, prostate, soy: may be associated with a reduction in risk.
- Menopause, red clover (*Trifolium pratense*): small effect for treating hot flushes.
- Menopause: seems to improve bone mineral density.

😐 *Unknown effectiveness*
- Cancer, colorectal: may be associated with a lower risk yet data contradictory.
- Diabetes type 2, red clover (*Trifolium pratense*): positive effects on blood pressure and endothelial function in postmenopausal women yet not enough data available.
- Diabetes type 2, soy: beneficial effects for fasting insulin, insulin resistance, total and LDL cholesterol yet not enough data available.
- Lipid profiles, sesame (*Sesamum indicum*) seed: not enough data available.
- Memory enhancement, cognitive performance: not enough data available.
- Menopause, flaxseed (*Linum usitatissimum*): not enough data available for treating hot flushes.
- Menopause, soy: contradictory and scarce data for symptom improvement including hot flushes and improving immune function.
- Menstrual migraine: not enough data available.
- Osteoporosis: data contradictory for measures of bone turnover and bone mineral density.
- Pregnancy rates: not enough data available.
- Premenstrual syndrome, soy: not enough data available.

☹ *Unlikely to be beneficial*
- Arthritis, psoriatic: no relevant effect for soy or seal oil.
- Body weight reduction: unlikely to be beneficial.
- Hypertension, soy: no meaningful effects.
- Lipid profiles, flaxseed *(Linum usitatissimum)*: unlikely to be beneficial.

✖ *Likely to be ineffective or harmful*
- Allergy and food intolerance: no effect for prevention in infants at high risk.
- Hypercholesterolaemia, red clover *(Trifolium pratense)*: likely to be ineffective for post-menopausal women.

Table 4.21 Systematic up-to-date reviews where phytoestrogens has been found to be beneficial

Condition	Source	No. of trials/ patients	Original conclusion
Lipid profiles	*Am J Cardiol* 2006; **98**:633–40	N=41/n=not available	[...] soy protein supplementation reduces serum lipids among adults with or without hypercholesterolemia.

Risks
- *Contraindications:* none known for phytoestrogens consumed as part of diet. Concentrated isoflavone supplements should not be taken during pregnancy or lactation, by children, or those with hormone-dependent tumours.
- *Precautions/warnings:* may affect the menstrual cycle. Possible proliferative effects on the endometrium, although data contradictory.
- *Adverse effects:* flatulence. For red clover, the limited evidence indicates no serious safety concerns associated with short-term use. No long-term safety data available.
- *Interactions:* none known.

Conclusions

- Soy reduces total cholesterol, LDL cholesterol and triglyceride levels and increases HDL; it might reduce the risk of breast and prostate cancer. Red clover may reduce hot flushes
- Few risks are reported for short-term use
- The risk-benefit profile is favourable for improving lipid profiles

Further reading

Cassidy A, Hooper L. Phytoestrogens and cardiovascular disease. *J Br Menopause Soc* 2006; **12**:49–56.
Nedrow A, Miller J, Walker M et al. Complementary and alternative therapies for the management of menopause-related symptoms: a systematic evidence review. *Arch Intern Med* 2006; **166**:1453–65.
Usui T. Pharmaceutical prospects of phytoestrogens. *Endocr J* 2006; **53**:7–20.

Probiotics

Profile

Origin
Probiotics are dietary supplements containing potentially beneficial bacteria or yeast and are intended to assist the body's naturally occurring gut flora to reestablish itself after for instance antibiotic therapy.

Main constituents
Lactic acid bacteria are one of the most commonly used probiotics.

Pharmacologic action
Anti-diarrhoeal.

Commonly used dosage
Depending on specific probiotic used.

Clinical bottom line
The data are based on systematic reviews only.

Benefits
:☺: *Beneficial*
- Diarrhoea, traveller's: beneficial for prevention.
- Diarrhoea, antibiotic-associated: beneficial for prevention (*Saccharomyces boulardii, Lactobacillus rhamnosus* GG).
- Diarrhoea, paediatric acute: beneficial for prevention.

☺ *Likely to be beneficial*
- Atopic dermatitis: may reduce severity and may prevent the condition.
- *Helicobacter pylori* infection: seems to be helpful in eradication therapy.
- Irritable bowel syndrome (*Lactobacillus plantarum*): seems to be helpful for global improvement of symptoms.
- Ulcerative colitis (*Bifidobacteria, Escherichia coli*): seem to reduce disease activity, prevent exacerbation and maintain remission.

☹ *Unknown effectiveness*
- Cholesterol reduction (*Bifodobacterium longum* BL 1): may reduce total and LDL-cholesterol yet not enough data available.
- Collagenous colitis: may improve symptoms yet not enough data available.
- Constipation (*Lactobacillus casei*): improvement in severity and stool consistency but not enough data available.
- Fatty liver disease, non-alcoholic: not enough data available.
- Irritable bowel syndrome: some positive effects reported for *Bifidobacterium infantis, Propionibacterium*, Prescript-Assist® and VSL 3®, yet not enough data available.
- Labour: not enough data available for preventing pre-term labour.
- Ulcerative colitis: not enough data available for *Lactobacillus* GG and VSL 3®.
- Urinary tract infection: not enough data available.

☹ *Unlikely to be beneficial*
- Lactose intolerance: seems to be ineffective for alleviating signs and symptoms.
- Probiotic (*Lactobacillus reuteri*, Medilac DS®, *Bacillus subtilis*, *Streptococcus faecium*): no effects for symptom improvement and quality of life.

✖ *Likely to be ineffective or harmful*
- Constipation (*Lactobacillus GG*): no improvement in spontaneous bowel movements.
- Crohn's disease: *Lactobacillus GG* and *Lactobacillus johnsonii LA1* seem to be ineffective for maintaining remission.
- Diarrhoea, associated with AIDS/HIV: no evidence of effectiveness

Table 4.22 Systematic up-to-date reviews where probiotics have been found to be beneficial

Condition	Source	No. of trials/ patients	Original conclusion
Traveller's diarrhoea	*Travel Med Infect Dis* 2007; **5**:97–105	N=12/n=not available	Several probiotics (*Saccharomyces boulardii* and a mixture of *Lactobacillus acidophilus* and *Bifidobacterium bifidum*) had significant efficacy. No serious adverse reactions were reported in the 12 trials
Antibiotic-associated diarrhoea	*Lancet Infect Dis* 2006; **6**:374–82	N=19/n=2038	The available data from the medical literature provides sufficient evidence for the role of probiotics in the prevention of acute diarrhoea
Paediatric acute diarrhoea	*Lancet Infect Dis* 2006; **6**:374–82	N=12/n=3197	Although higher in children, the effect of probiotics is also observed in adults. The effect on antibiotic-associated diarrhoea is most pronounced, but is also observed in non-antibiotic-associated diarrhoea and non-travellers' diarrhoea

Risks
- *Contraindications:* pregnancy and lactation.
- *Precautions/warnings:* none.
- *Adverse effects:* diarrhoea, bloating, flatulence, constipation.
- *Interactions:* none.

Conclusions

- Probiotics are beneficial for acute diarrhoea such as traveller's diarrhoea, antibiotic-associated diarrhoea, and paediatric acute diarrhoea; they are likely to be beneficial for atopic dermatitis, *H. pylori* infection, irritable bowel syndrome and ulcerative colitis
- Adverse events seem rare
- The risk–benefit for diarrhoea is positive and likely to be positive for the above conditions

Further reading

Parkes GC. An overview of probiotics and prebiotics. *Nurs Stand* 2007; **21**:43–7.

Propolis

Profile

Origin

A resinous material made by bees, produced by combining resin from the buds of various trees with other substances such as salivary secretions and beewax.

Main constituents

Flavonoids, hydroxycinnammic acids.

Pharmacologic action

Antimicrobial, anti-inflammatory, antioxidant, cytotoxic.

Commonly used dosage

Mouthwash: once or twice daily.

Clinical bottom line

Benefits

😐 *Unknown effectiveness*

- Acute uterine cervicitis: not enough data available.
- Aphthous stomatitis: may reduce outbreak frequency but not enough data available.
- Asthma, reduction in attacks: yet not enough data available.
- Cervical dysplasia: may help reduce human papillomavirus infection yet few data available.
- Dental plaque reduction: not enough data available.
- Herpes genitalis: faster average healing time and reduced incidence of superinfection, not enough data available.
- Herpes labialis recurrences: not enough data available.
- Respiratory tract infections: not enough data available.

😟 *Unlikely to be beneficial*

- Crohn's disease.
- Ulcerative colitis.

Risks

- *Contraindications:* allergy to bee stings.
- *Precautions/warnings:* other allergic predispositions.
- *Adverse effects:* allergic reactions, contact dermatitis, hyperkeratotic dermatitis, vesicular dermatitis, itching, swelling, mucositis, stomatitis.
- *Interactions:* none known.

Conclusions

- The evidence for propolis is not convincing for any condition
- Propolis seems relatively safe although allergic reactions have been reported
- The risk–benefit balance fails to be positive. Considering the costs involved and the availability of other conventional treatment approaches, these might be preferred

Further reading

Castaldo S, Capasso F. Propolis, an old remedy used in modern medicine. *Fitoterapia* 2002; **73**:S1–6.
Khalil ML. Biological activity of bee propolis in health and disease. *Asian Pac J Cancer Prev* 2006; 7:22–31.

Psyllium (*Plantago ovata*)

Profile

Origin

Psyllium is an annual herb that grows to a height of 30–46 cm. *Plantaga ovata* and *P. psyllium* are produced commercially in several European and other countries particularly India. Mucilage, a fibrous, hydrophilic material, is obtained from its seed coat. It absorbs excess water while stimulating normal bowel elimination.

Main constituents

Polysaccharides, fatty acids.

Pharmacologic action

Antihypercholesterolaemic, antiglycaemic, laxative.

Commonly used dosage

5–15g daily.

Clinical bottom line

Benefits

😊 *Beneficial*
- Constipation, chronic: evidence supports its use.

😊 *Likely to be beneficial*
- Diabetes, type 2: seems to reduce fasting plasma glucose, total, and LDL cholesterol.
- Hypercholesterolaemia: causes a modest reduction in total and LDL cholesterol.
- Irritable bowel syndrome: seems to improve global symptoms.
- Ulcerative colitis: seems to improve symptoms and maintain patients in remission.

😐 *Unknown effectiveness*
- Diarrhoea: may improve urgency and stool consistency: may reduce incidence and severity of radiation-induced diarrhoea in cancer patients.
- Hypertension: may reduce blood pressure but not enough data available.
- Parkinson's disease: may increase stool frequency yet not enough data available.

😟 *Unlikely to be beneficial*
- Body weight reduction: data indicate no beneficial effects.

Risks
- *Contraindications:* pregnancy and lactation, bowel obstruction.
- *Precautions/warnings:* none.
- *Adverse effects:* allergic reactions including anaphylaxis.
- *Interactions:* increased effects of cardiac glycosides, may increase effects of diabetic medication.

Conclusions

- Psyllium is effective in improving constipation; it is likely to be beneficial for diabetes, irritable bowel syndrome, ulcerative colitis, and in lowering total and LDL cholesterol levels in patients with hypercholesterolaemia
- Adverse events such as allergic reactions including anaphylaxis were reported but seem rare
- The risk–benefit balance is positive for constipation and likely to be positive for diabetes, hypercholesterolaemia, irritable bowel syndrome and ulcerative colitis

Further reading

Petchetti L, Frishman WH, Petrillo R, Raju K. Nutriceuticals in cardiovascular disease: psyllium. *Cardiol Rev* 2007; **15**:116–22.

Pumpkin (*Cucurbita pepo*)

Profile

Origin
Pumpkin is a squash fruit that grows from a trailing vine of the genus *Cucurbita*. The seeds of pumpkins are used medicinally.

Main constituents
Cucurbitin, sterols, minerals, vitamins, fatty acids.

Presumed pharmacologic action
Antiandrogenic, anti-inflammatory.

Commonly used dosage
480mg daily of seed extract.

Clinical bottom line

Benefits

☹ *Unknown effectiveness*
- Benign prostatic hyperplasia: may have positive effects on urinary symptoms yet not enough data available.

Risks
- *Contraindications:* pregnancy and lactation.
- *Precautions/warnings:* none known.
- *Adverse effects:* none known.
- *Interactions:* none known.

Conclusions

- Data suggest that there is no convincing evidence of effectiveness
- Adverse events seem to be rare
- The risk–benefit ratio fails to be positive for any condition

Red clover (*Trifolium pratense*)

Profile

Origin
A plant that is native to most European countries and has a long history of medicinal use. Flower heads are employed for medicinal purposes.

Main constituents
Coumarins, isoflavonoids, saponins, volatile oil.

Presumed pharmacologic action
Oestrogenic.

Commonly used dosage
Extract containing 40–160mg isoflavones per day.

Clinical bottom line

Benefits

😊 *Likely to be beneficial*
- Menopause: small reduction of the frequency of hot flushes.

😐 *Unknown effectiveness*
- Cancer, breast or endometrial, protection: not enough data available.
- Cardiovascular risk factors: normalization of blood lipids, blood pressure, arterial stiffness, not enough data available.
- Menopause: osteoporosis or cyclical mastalgia, not enough data available.

Table 4.23 Systematic up-to-date review where red clover has been found likely to be beneficial

Condition	Source	No. of trials/ patients	Original conclusion
Menopausal symptoms	*Phytomedicine* 2007; **14**:153-9	N=11/n=1160	There is evidence of a marginally significant effect … for treating hot flushes in menopausal women

Risks
- *Contraindications:* pregnancy and lactation.
- *Precautions/warnings:* hormone-sensitive cancers, coagulation abnormalities.
- *Adverse effects:* allergic reactions, breast tenderness, alterations of menstruations, weight gain.
- *Interactions:* anticoagulants, hormonal drugs, tamoxifen, increase of blood levels of drugs metabolized by cytochrome P450 enzymes.

Conclusions

- Reduces menopausal hot flushes but the effect size is modest
- Some risks are known
- The risk–benefit balance may be positive for treatment of hot flushes provided that risks are adequately managed

Red yeast rice (*Monascus purpureus*)

Profile

Origin

Red yeast rice is the product of fermenting rice with *Monascus purpureus* yeast.

Main constituents

Lovastatin, mevinic acids, sterols, isoflavones.

Presumed pharmacologic action

Blockage of cholesterol biosynthesis, anti-inflammatory.

Commonly used dosage

1200mg twice daily.

Clinical bottom line

Benefits

😊 *Likely to be beneficial*

- Hypercholesterolaemia: may reduce total, LDL cholesterol and triglyceride levels but some studies are flawed.

Risks

- *Contraindications:* pregnancy, liver disease, thyroid disease.
- *Precautions/warnings:* lactation.
- *Adverse effects:* gastrointestinal symptoms, liver damage, heartburn, dizziness.
- *Interactions:* other cholesterol-lowering drugs, grapefruit juice.

Conclusions

- Cholesterol-lowering effects are well-documented
- Serious risks have been noted, but seem to be rare
- The risk–benefit balance is not entirely convincing but seems to be similar to that of lovastatin

Further reading

Liu J, Zhang J, Shi Y, Grimsgaard S *et al.* Chinese red yeast rice (*Monascus purpureus*) for primary hyperlipidemia: a meta-analysis of randomized controlled trials. *Chin Med* 2006; **1**:4.

S-adenosyl-L-methionine (SAM-e)

Profile

Origin
Molecule that is produced from methionine and adenosine triphosphate in most cells of the body.

Presumed pharmacologic action
SAM-e participates in many biological processes. It has a short half-life and low levels of it are claimed to be the cause of a wide range of conditions. SAM-e is alleged to have analgetic and inflammatory activity.

Commonly used dosage
- Oral: 400–1600mg/day.
- Intravenous or intramuscular injections: 200–400mg/day.

Clinical bottom line

Benefits
😊 Beneficial
- Osteoarthritis: improves pain and function.

😐 Unknown effectiveness
- Alcoholic liver disease: trial data methodologically weak.
- Fibromyalgia, pain: data contradictory.
- Migraine, frequency of attacks: not enough data available.

Table 4.24 Systematic up-to-date reviews where SAM-e has been found to be beneficial

Treatment	Source	No. of trials/ patients	Original conclusion
Osteoarthritis	J Fam Pract 2002; **51**:425–30	N=11/n=1442	SAM-e appears to be as effective as NSAIDs in reducing pain and improving functional limitations

Risks
- Contraindications: pregnancy and lactation.
- Precautions/warnings: depression.
- Adverse effects: vomiting, gastrointestinal symptoms, headache.
- Interactions: none known.

Conclusions

- SAM-e improves function and reduces pain of osteoarthritis
- Only minor risks are on record
- The risk–benefit balance is positive for osteoarthritis
- SAM-e could be used as an adjunct to conventional treatments for osteoarthritis

Saw palmetto (*Serenoa repens*)

Profile

Origin

A dwarf palm, the fruits are used for medicinal purposes. Commercially available preparations contain the lipophilic fraction, extracted with hexane or liquid carbon dioxide.

Main constituents

Fatty acids, flavonoids, phytosterols, and polysaccharides.

Presumed pharmacologic action

Inhibition of 5-alpha-reductase, inhibitory effects on the binding of dihydrotestosterone to androgen receptors in the prostate: anti-inflammatory, antiproliferative prolactin inhibition.

Commonly used dosage

Typically, 320mg of liposterolic extract daily in divided doses.

Clinical bottom line

Benefits

🙂 *Beneficial*

- Benign prostatic hyperplasia: mild-to-moderate improvement in urinary symptoms and flow measures.

😐 *Unknown effectiveness*

- Androgenic alopecia: encouraging yet insufficient evidence.

😠 *Unlikely to be beneficial*

- Prostatitis/chronic pelvic pain: no improvements reported after 1-year treatment period.

Table 4.25 Systematic up-to-date review where saw palmetto has been found to be beneficial

Condition	Source	No. of trials/ patients	Original conclusion
Benign prostatic hyperplasia	*Cochrane Database Syst Rev* 2002; **3**:CD001423	N=21/n=3139	The evidence suggests that *Serenoa repens* provides mild to moderate improvement in urinary symptoms and flow measures. *S. repens* produced similar improvement in urinary symptoms and flow compared to finasteride and is associated with fewer adverse treatment events

Risks
- *Contraindications:* pregnancy and lactation.
- *Precautions/warnings:* allergy or hypersensitivity, may increase bleeding time.
- *Adverse effects:* gastrointestinal complaints, bleeding, haemorrhage, dizziness, headache, constipation, diarrhoea, dysuria.
- *Interactions:* hormone replacement therapy, oral contraceptives, may increase the effects of antiandrogenic drugs, and decrease the effects of androgenic drugs. Minimal risk for cytochrome P450-mediated herb-drug interactions in humans.

Conclusions

- Improves urinary symptoms and flow measures of benign prostatic hyperplasia
- Encouraging safety profile
- Positive risk–benefit balance for treating benign prostatic hyperplasia
- Improvement of symptoms and objective signs of benign prostatic hyperplasia possibly to the same extent as with finasteride

Further reading

Ulbricht C, Basch E, Bent S *et al.* Evidence-based systematic review of saw palmetto by the Natural Standard Research Collaboration. *J Soc Integr Oncol* 2006; **4**:170–86.

Shark cartilage

Profile

Origin

Shark cartilage capsules contain dried and powdered cartilage from the fins of the hammerhead shark (*Sphyrna lewini*) or the spiny dogfish shark (*Squalus acanthias*).

Main constituents

Sphyrastatin1 and sphyrastatin2.

Presumed pharmacologic action

Antiangiogenic.

Commonly used dosage

500–4500mg daily.

Clinical bottom line

Benefits

☒ *Likely to be ineffective or harmful*
- Cancer: does not increase survival rates or improve quality of life.

Risks

- *Contraindications:* pregnancy and lactation.
- *Precautions/warnings:* liver diseases.
- *Adverse effects:* hepatitis, hyper- and hypoglycaemia, generalized weakness, peripheral oedema.
- *Interactions:* none known.

Conclusions

- The best clinical trials suggest no effectiveness for cancer
- Several serious adverse effects are on record
- The risk–benefit balance is clearly negative
- Shark cartilage use should be discouraged

Further reading

Gonzalez RP, Leyva A, Moraes MO. Shark cartilage as source of antiangiogenic compounds: from basic to clinical research. *Biol Pharm Bull* 2001; **24**:1097–101.

St John's wort (*Hypericum perforatum*)

Profile

Origin

Aerial parts of this common plant are used. Its name is said to originate from John the Baptist.

Main constituents

Hypericin, hyperforin.

Presumed pharmacologic action

Selective serotonin re-uptake inhibitor, monoamine oxidase inhibitor, antiviral activity.

Commonly used dosage

900mg per day, in divided doses, of extract standardized to 0.3% hypericin or 5% hyperforin.

Clinical bottom line

Benefits

☺ *Beneficial*

- Depression: beneficial for mild-to-moderate forms of depression, several positive meta-analyses are available.

☺ *Unknown effectiveness*

- Atopic dermatitis: topical, not enough data available.
- Major depression: results conflicting.
- Seasonal affective disorder: not enough data available.
- Somatoform disorders: not enough data available.

☒ *Likely to be ineffective or harmful*

- HIV/AIDS: no evidence of antiviral activity.
- Obsessive compulsive disorder: no evidence of effectiveness.
- Premenstrual syndrome: no evidence of effectiveness.
- Social phobia: no evidence of effectiveness.
- Smoking cessation: not enough data, preliminary results are not encouraging.

Table 4.26 Systematic up-to-date review where St John's wort has been found to be beneficial

Treatment	Source	No. of trials/ patients	Original conclusion
Depression	*Fortschr Neurol Psychiatr* 2004; **72**:330–43	N=30/n=NA	St John's wort is effective for mild to moderate depression

Risks

- *Contraindications:* pregnancy and lactation.
- *Precautions/warnings:* photosensitization.
- *Adverse effects:* allergic reaction, gastrointestinal symptoms, fatigue, mania.
- *Interactions:* conventional antidepressants, drug metabolized by cytochrome P450 enzymes.

Conclusions

- Effective for mild-to-moderate depression
- Some risks exist, particularly interactions
- The risk–benefit balance can be positive provided risks are adequately managed
- St John's wort can be a useful alternative to synthetic antidepressants in treating mild to moderate depression

Further reading

Werneke U, Turner T, Priebe S. Complementary medicines in psychiatry: review of effectiveness and safety. *Br J Psychiatry* 2006; **188**:109–21.

Linde K, Mulrow CD, Berner M, Egger M. St John's wort for depression. Cochrane Database Syst Rev 2005; **2**: CD000448.

Tea tree (*Melaleuca alternifolia*)

Profile

Origin

Leaves and branches are used for extraction of their essential oils. Commonly contained in modern cosmetics.

Main constituents

Cineole, pinene, symene (and many other compounds).

Presumed pharmacologic action

Antimicrobial.

Commonly used dosage

5–100% oil for topical application several times daily.

Clinical bottom line

Benefits

😑 *Unknown effectiveness*

- Acne, control of skin lesions: not enough data available.
- Athlete's foot (tinea pedis), control of infection: not enough data available.
- Candidiasis of patients with AIDS: not enough data available.
- Chronic gingivitis, control of inflammation: not enough data available.
- Fungal infections, other, control of infection: not enough data available.
- Onychomycosis, control of infection: not enough data available.
- *Staphylococcus aureus* infection: not enough data available.

😣 *Unlikely to be beneficial*

- Herpes labialis: not effective in the treatment of recurrent herpes labialis.

Risks

- *Contraindications:* allergy to tea tree oil, pregnancy and lactation.
- *Precautions/warnings:* not for internal use, not for topical use on mucous membranes or injured skin.
- *Adverse effects:* allergic reactions are frequent, skin irritation.
- *Interactions:* none known.

Conclusions

- Effectiveness not proven for any indication
- Some risks, predominantly allergic reactions
- The risk–benefit balance fails to be positive
- For the conditions in question conventional treatments are usually highly effective and tea tree oil has little to offer in addition

Further reading

Carson CF, Hammer KA, Riley TV. *Melaleuca alternifolia* (tea tree) oil: a review of antimicrobial and other medicinal properties. *Clin Microbiol Rev* 2006; **19**:50–62.

Thunder god vine (*Tripterygium wilfordii*)

Profile

Origin

Plant used frequently in traditional Chinese medicine: the roots are used for medicinal purposes. Water decoctions proved toxic; ethyl acetate or chloroform-methanol extracts supposedly overcome this problem.

Main constituents

Triterpenoids, triptolide.

Presumed pharmacologic action

Immunosuppression, inhibition of cytokine-production, antifertility effect in men, antiviral, antitumour.

Commonly used dosage

180–360mg extract per day.

Clinical bottom line

Benefits

🕮 *Trade off between benefits and harms:*
- Rheumatoid arthritis: positive data for pain and function but it is associated with considerable risks.

☒ *Likely to be ineffective or harmful*
- Allograft rejection in patients after kidney transplant: preliminary data positive but associated with considerable risks.
- Graves's opthalmopathy: preliminary data are encouraging but it is associated with considerable risks.
- Male contraception: preliminary data encouraging but associated with considerable risks.

Table 4.27 Systematic up-to-date review where thunder god vine has been found to be effective

Condition	Source	No. of trials/ patients	Original conclusion
Rheumatoid arthritis	*Phytomedicine* 2006; **13**:371–7	N=2/n=105	*T. wilfordii* has beneficial effects on the symptoms of RA. However, the literature indicates that *T. wilfordii* is associated with serious adverse events which make the risk–benefit analysis for this herb unfavourable

Risks

- *Contraindications:* pregnancy (teratogenic effects).
- *Precautions/warnings:* lactation (insufficient information).
- *Adverse effects:* predisposition to infection, dysmenorrhoea, infertility, gastrointestinal symptoms, vomiting, diarrhoea, lymphocyte suppression, allergic reactions, impairment of renal function, hypertension, hypotension, shock.
- *Interactions:* effects of immunosuppressants can be enhanced.

Conclusions

- Effective in improving pain and function in rheumatoid arthritis
- Considerable risks are on record
- The risk–benefit balance fails to be positive for any condition

Thyme (*Thymus vulgaris, T. zygis*)

Profile

Origin
There are up to 400 subspecies of thyme: common thyme (*Thymus vulgaris*) and Spanish thyme (*T. zygis*) are often used interchangeably for medicinal purposes. Leaves and flowers are the parts used.

Main constituents
Camphene, eugenol, flavonoids, phenols (thymol, carvacrol), rosmarinic acid.

Presumed pharmacologic action
Antimicrobial, antitussive, spasmolytic and antioxidant.

Commonly used dosage
- Tea: 1–2g of dried herb in 150mL boiling water for 10 minutes.
- Liquid extract: 1–2g of extract in fluid/one cup water up to 3 times daily: 20–40 drops liquid extract (1:1 weight/volume fresh leaf or 1:4 dried leaf) 3 times daily in juice: 40 drops tincture (1:10 in 70% ethanol) up to 3 times daily.
- Oil: 2–3 drops thyme oil on a sugar cube 2–3 times daily has been used: thyme oil is considered to be highly toxic if undiluted.

Clinical bottom line

Benefits
No compelling trial evidence exists for thyme taken on its own.

😊 *Likely to be beneficial*
- Chronic bronchitis: encouraging results for a combination product with other herbs.

😐 *Unknown effectiveness*
- Dyspraxia: thyme oil in combination with evening primrose oil, fish oils, and vitamin E improved movement disorders in children but not enough data available.
- Hair loss/alopecia areata: topically applied thyme oil in combination with other essential oil improved hair growth yet not enough data available.

☠ *Likely to be ineffective or harmful*
- Eczema: aromatherapy massage with essential oils.

Risks
- *Contraindications:* pregnancy and lactation (emmenagogue and abortifacient), gastritis, enterocolitis, allergy to *Labiatae* family, congestive heart failure.
- *Precautions/warnings:* patients with gastrointestinal problems, thyroid disorders. Avoid oral ingestion or non-diluted application.
- *Adverse effects:* nausea, vomiting, diarrhea, headache, dizziness, respiratory distress, bradycardia, dermatitis (topical use).
- *Interactions:* none known.

Conclusions

- Thyme in combination products is likely to be effective for bronchitis compared to synthetic medications
- Generally well tolerated in recommended doses: the majority of adverse events appear to be related to dermatologic or allergic reactions
- The risk–benefit balance for a combination product is likely to be positive but the lack of data regarding thyme as a monotherapy prevents a conclusive evaluation

Further reading

Basch E, Ulbricht C, Hammerness P *et al.* Thyme (*Thymus vulgaris* L.), thymol. *J Herb Pharmacother* 2004; **4**:49–67.

Thymus extract

Profile

Origin

Bovine thymus gland. Purified, sterile extract is used for injection. Several commercial preparations are available.

Main constituents

Polypeptides.

Presumed pharmacologic action

Stimulation of immune response.

Commonly used dosage

Varies according to nature of extract.

Clinical bottom line

Benefits

😐 *Unknown effectiveness*

- Eczema: not enough data available.
- Hepatitis B: most trials positive but methodologically weak.
- Herpes simplex labialis recurrent infection: not enough data available.

😧 *Unlikely to be beneficial*

- Cancer: the most reliable trials do not suggest effectiveness.

Risks

- *Contraindications:* known hypersensitivity.
- *Precautions/warnings:* pregnancy, lactation.
- *Adverse effects:* allergic reactions, anaphylactic shock, transmission of infections.
- *Interactions:* other drugs affecting the immune system.

Conclusions

- The effectiveness of thymus therapy is not proven for any indication
- The risks of injecting bovine peptides can be considerable
- The risk–benefit balance for thymus extracts fails to be positive

Turmeric (*Curcuma longa*)

Profile

Origin

Turmeric is a member of the ginger family, *Zingiberaceae*. The rhizome is used in traditional Asian medicine and also as a deep yellow spice in curries and other South Asian cuisine. It is also used to protect food products from sunlight and coded as E100 when used as a food additive.

Main constituents

Curcumin.

Presumed pharmacologic action

Antiseptic, anti-inflammatory, antioxidant.

Commonly used dosage

2g turmeric daily in four divided doses.

Clinical bottom line

Benefits

😐 *Unknown effectiveness*

- Anterior uveitis: may improve symptoms yet not enough data available.
- Biliary dyskinesia: a combination preparation (Cholagogum F) may reduce colic pain.
- Depression: a combination preparation may improve Hamilton Depression scores.
- Irritable bowel syndrome: may improve quality of life yet not enough data available.
- Knee surgery: a combination preparation may reduce pain and swelling.
- Non-ulcer dyspepsia: not enough data available.
- Osteoarthritis, knee: as part of a combination preparation (RA-11) may reduce pain severity.
- Pancreatitis, tropical: a combination of curcumin and piperine may reverse lipid peroxidation.
- Ulcerative colitis: may reduce relapse rates yet not enough data available.
- Vaginal infections: a combination preparation may improve smear tests.

😣 *Unlikely to be beneficial*

- Irritable bowel syndrome: *C. xanthorrhiza* seems unlikely to be beneficial.
- Obesity: a combination preparation has no effects on weight loss.

Risks

- *Contraindications:* pregnancy and lactation.
- *Precautions/warnings:* may increase the risk of bleeding, allergic reactions.
- *Adverse effects:* gastrointestinal complaints, heartburn, nausea, diarrhoea.
- *Interactions:* aspirin, anticoagulants, NSAIDs drugs.

Conclusions

- Data suggest that the evidence is not convincing for any condition
- Adverse events are on record
- The risk–benefit ratio fails to be positive for any condition

Valerian (*Valeriana officinalis, V. edulis*)

Profile

Origin
For medicinal purposes, the rhizomes of *V. officinalis* and *V. edulis* are used.

Main constituents
Valepotriates, alkaloids, amino acids, volatile oils.

Presumed pharmacologic action
Sedative, anxiolytic possibly involving gamma-aminobutyric acid (GABA) receptors.

Commonly used dosage
400–900mg extract before bedtime.

Clinical bottom line

Benefits

☺ *Likely to be beneficial*
- Insomnia, sleep latency/quality: data positive but evidence is somewhat contradictory

☹ *Unknown effectiveness*
- Withdrawal symptoms, benzodiazepines: not enough data available.

✖ *Likely to be ineffective or harmful*
- Anxiety: efficacy has not been demonstrated.

Table 4.28 Systematic up-to-date reviews where valerian has been found likely to be beneficial

Treatment	Source	No. of trials/ patients	Original conclusion
Insomnia	*Am J Med* 2006; **119**:1005–12	N=16/n=1093	Valerian might improve sleep quality

Risks
- *Contraindications:* pregnancy and lactation, liver disease.
- *Precautions/warnings:* long-term usage, do not operate machinery after taking valerian.
- *Adverse effects:* liver damage has been associated with combination preparations.
- *Interactions:* may enhance the effects of sedatives, hypnotics and other drugs.

Conclusions

- Valerian is likely to be an effective herbal 'sleeping pill'
- Mostly minor risks reported
- The risk–benefit balance is likely to be positive
- There are, of course, effective treatments for insomnia but, in case patients prefer a herbal option, valerian might be worth trying

Further reading

Miyasaka LS, Atallah AN, Soares BG. Valerian for anxiety disorders. *Cochrane Database Syst Rev* 2006; **4**:CD004515.

Willow (*Salix* spp)

Profile

Origin
The bark of the willow tree has been traditionally used as a remedy for inflammatory joint diseases and was later rediscovered as a remedy for fever and pain. Salicin was isolated as an active compound and became aspirin.

Main constituents
Derivatives of salicin, mainly salicortin, tannins, tremulacin.

Presumed pharmacologic action
Salicin is metabolized to salicylic acid which has antipyretic and analgesic effects.

Commonly used dosage
120–240mg of total salicin daily in divided doses.

Clinical bottom line

Benefits

☺ *Likely to be beneficial*
- Low back pain, non-specific: short-term pain improvements for willow.

☹ *Unknown effectiveness*
- Osteoarthritis, pain: not enough data available.
- Migraine, prophylaxis: not enough data available.

☹ *Unlikely to be beneficial*
- Rheumatoid arthritis: no improvement in pain.

Table 4.29 Systematic up-to-date review where willow has been found likely to be beneficial

Condition	Source	No. of trials/ patients	Original conclusion
Low back pain, non-specific	*Cochrane Database Syst Rev* 2006; **2**: CD004504	N=3/n=470	An extract of *Salix alba* at a standardized dosage of 240mg salicin/day seems to reduce pain more than placebo

Risks
- *Contraindications:* pregnancy and lactation, patients with salicylate intolerance.
- *Precautions/warnings:* patients on anticoagulation treatment should use willow bark extracts only under careful supervision.
- *Adverse effects:* anaphylactic reactions, gastrointestinal complaints, skin rashes.
- *Interactions:* additive effects on anticoagulants and other salicylate containing drugs.

Conclusions

- Willow extract is likely to be beneficial for episodes of chronic low-back pain
- The adverse events profile is favourable if precautions are regarded
- The risk–benefit balance seems positive but not entirely convincing

Yohimbe (*Pausinystalia johimbe*)

Profile

Origin
A tall evergreen tree, native to Central Africa. The ground bark is traditionally used as an aphrodisiac, particularly for male erectile dysfunction. Yohimbine is the main active constituent of yohimbe bark extract. Most clinical studies relate to the effects of this isolated constituent.

Main constituents
Indole alkaloids of which 10–15% are yohimbine.

Presumed pharmacologic action
Alpha-2-adrenoceptor blockade. Rise in sympathetic drive by increasing noradrenaline release and firing rate of noradrenergic nuclei in the central nervous system.

Commonly used dosage
16–18mg of yohimbine hydrochloride daily in divided doses.

Clinical bottom line

Benefits
:☺: *Beneficial*
- Erectile dysfunction: organic or nonorganic causes.

☺ *Unknown effectiveness*
- Dry mouth in patients receiving psychotropic drugs: not enough data available.
- Hypotension, orthostatic in Parkinson's disease: not enough data available.
- Major depressive disorder: as an addition to fluoxetine, not enough data available.
- Overweight/obesity: conflicting results for body weight reduction, more data required.
- Sexual dysfunction, pre/postmenopausal women: conflicting results.
- Withdrawal symptoms due to drug abuse: not enough data available.

Risks
- *Contraindications:* pregnancy and lactation, children, known allergy to yohimbe, psychiatric conditions, use of phenothiazine-containing agents, sympathomimetic agents.
- *Precautions/warnings:* individuals with chronic inflammation of the prostate or the reproductive organs, anxiety disorders, hypertension, cardiac, renal or hepatic diseases.
- *Adverse effects:* nervous excitation, tremor, irritability, sleeplessness, anxiety, hypertension, hypotension, tachycardia, bronchospasm, gastrointestinal complaints, skin flushing, rash, mydriasis.
- *Interactions:* increased effects of antidepressants, central nervous system stimulants, phenothiazines and other alpha2-adrenoceptor blocking agents, reduced effects of antihypertensive drugs, benzodiazepines: interaction with sildenafil is theoretically possible.

Conclusions

- There is little evidence for the effectiveness and safety of yohimbe bark extract. The evidence relates mostly to its isolated main constituent yohimbine, which has beneficial effects in the treatment of erectile dysfunction of various causes
- Advantages over invasive interventions exist, and in this scenario relatively safer
- The risk–benefit balance seems favourable for erectile dysfunction

Further reading

Crassous PA, Denis C, Paris H, Senard JM. Interest of alpha2-adrenergic agonists and antagonists in clinical practice: background, facts and perspectives. *Curr Top Med Chem* 2007; **7**:187–94.
Tam SW, Worcel M, Wyllie M. Yohimbine: a clinical review. *Pharmacol Ther* 2001; **91**:215–43.

Chapter 5

Conditions

Cardiology

Angina (pectoris)

Profile

Myocardial ischaemia, often experienced as tightness of the chest, discomfort in the chest, shoulder, back arm, or jaw. Its cause is usually coronary heart disease, i.e. arteriosclerotic narrowing of the arteries supplying the heart. Less frequently it is due to coronary spasms. Angina is often characterized as stable (regular or predictable symptoms) and unstable (rapid symptomatic decline, pain at rest signalling plaque instability). Any type of angina is a serious symptom often followed by myocardial infarction. Around 10–15% of people over the age of 65 experience angina. Risk factor elimination is the best prevention. CAM is used frequently, particularly supplements.

Clinical bottom line

:☻: *Beneficial*

- Relaxation: as an adjunct to conventional treatments, it improves exercise tolerance and reduces pain.

☻ *Likely to be beneficial*

- Acupuncture: preliminary data suggest pain reduction.

☹ *Unknown effectiveness*

- Abana (Ayurvedic herbal preparation): not enough data available.
- Chinese herbal mixtures: many mixtures exist and for any one preparation the evidence is unconvincing.
- Homeopathy: not enough data available.
- Pomegranate (*Punica granatum*): not enough data available.
- *Terminalia arjuna*: not enough data available.

☹ *Unlikely to be beneficial*

- Chelation therapy: the most rigorous studies fail to show effectiveness.

🐾 *Likely to be ineffective or harmful*

- Fish oil: no effect on angina symptoms.

Table 5.1 Systematic up-to-date reviews of treatments that are beneficial for angina

Treatment	Source	No. of trials/ patients	Original conclusion
Relaxation	*Eur J Cardiovasc Prev Rehabil* 2005; **12**:193–202	N=27/n=2181	Intensive supervised relaxation practice enhances recovery from an ischaemic cardiac event and contributes to secondary prevention. It is an important ingredient of cardiac rehabilitation, in addition to exercise and psycho-education

Conclusions

- Relaxation is beneficial as an adjunct to conventional care; acupuncture is likely to be helpful for reducing symptoms
- Both of these options are not associated with frequent, serious harm
- The risk–benefit balance for relaxation is positive; for acupuncture it is probably positive
- Conventional treatments for angina are usually very effective. Therefore CAM is merely an adjunct to it

Further reading

Natarajan M. Angina (unstable). *Clin Evid* 2005; **14**:60–70.

Relaxation therapy

What is it?
Techniques for eliciting the 'relaxation response' of the autonomic nervous system

How does it work?
Progressive muscle relaxation elicits the relaxation response, resulting in the normalizing of blood supply to the muscles, decreases in oxygen consumption, heart rate, respiration and skeletal muscle activity and increases in skin resistance and alpha brain waves. Other relaxation techniques involve passive muscle relaxation, refocusing, or breathing

How is it used?
Several months of daily practice is needed in order to be able to evoke the relaxation response

Are there any risks?
None known

Chronic heart failure

Profile

Heart failure (synonym cardiac failure) occurs when abnormal cardiac function causes failure of the heart to pump blood at a rate sufficient for metabolic requirements. It can be caused by systolic or diastolic dysfunction and is associated with neurohormonal changes. Signs and symptoms of chronic heart failure (CHF) can include fatigue and weakness, dyspnoea, reduced ability to exercise, persistent cough or wheezing, oedema in legs, ankles, and feet. Heart failure often develops after other cardiac conditions have damaged the heart. Risk factors of CHF such as smoking, obesity, or diet high in cholesterol and/or fat may contribute to heart failure. CAM modalities most frequently recommended for CHF are herbal and nonherbal dietary supplements.

Clinical bottom line

☺ Beneficial

- Hawthorn (*Crataegus* spp): improvements in maximal workload with extracts from leaf and flower.

☺ Likely to be beneficial

- Milk vetch (*Astragalus* spp): improvements in left ventricular ejection fraction.

☻ Unknown effectiveness

- Acupuncture: not enough data available.
- Ayurvedic medicines: not enough data available.
- Chinese medicines: not enough data available.
- Co-enzyme Q10: contradictory findings and methodological weaknesses.
- Ginseng (*Panax ginseng*): not enough data available.
- Kanlijian: increases walking distance and quality of life but not enough data available.
- Meditation: improvement in quality of life but not enough data available.
- Micronutrients: increases in left ventricular ejection fraction but not enough data available.
- MyoVive: not enough data available.
- Relaxation: improvement in quality of life but not enough data available.
- Vitamin D: reduces inflammatory milieu.

☒ Likely to be ineffective or harmful

- Vitamin E: likely to be ineffective.

Conclusions

- Best evidence supports the use of hawthorn extract. Milk vetch is likely to be beneficial for improving left ventricular ejection fraction
- Hawthorn and milk vetch are not associated with serious risks but allergic reactions must be considered
- The risk–benefit balance for hawthorn is clearly positive for mild-to-moderate CHF. For milk vetch the risk–benefit balance is likely but not convincingly positive
- Hawthorn leaf and flower extract has been implied to be similarly effective as some conventional drugs

Further reading

Yeh GY, Davis RB, Phillips RS. Use of complementary therapies in patients with cardiovascular disease. *Am J Cardiol* 2006; **98**:673–80.

Hawthorn (*Crataegus spp*)

What is it?

Crataegus species found in hawthorn preparations include mainly *C. laevigata* and *C. monogyna*

How does it work?

Dilation of coronary arteries, positive inotropic, decrease of atrioventricular conduction time, and increase of refractory period, cardioprotective, anti-arrhythmic, hypotensive, beta-blocking and ACE-inhibiting activity, antioxidant. The mechanism of action is similar to digitalis

How is it used?

Orally as tablets or capsules

Are there any risks?

Nausea, dizziness, vertigo, fatigue, sweating, palpitations, tachycardia, and gastrointestinal complaints have been reported

Hypertension

Profile

Chronically elevated blood pressure (i.e. in excess of 140/90mmHg) is a common, well-documented, independent cardiovascular risk factor. Primary or essential hypertension has no known causes. Prevalence of hypertension is highly age-dependent with older people having higher blood pressure. Secondary hypertension is due to other diseases such as kidney disease or tumours, especially of the adrenal gland. Herbal remedies and biofeedback are used in particular.

Clinical bottom line

☺ Beneficial

- Biofeedback: lowers systolic and diastolic blood pressure.

☺ Likely to be beneficial

- Autogenic training: even though not all trials are of high quality, a positive effect seems likely.
- Co-enzyme Q10: small reductions of both systolic and diastolic pressures when administered with other antihypertensives.
- Fish oil: reductions of elevated diastolic and systolic pressures at high doses.
- Hibiscus (*Hibiscus sabdariffa*): seems to reduce diastolic blood pressure.
- Qigong: might lower systolic blood pressure.
- Relaxation: effect probably too small to be clinically relevant.
- Tai chi: seems to reduce systolic and diastolic blood pressure.
- Yoga: data encouraging but not fully convincing.

☺ Unknown effectiveness

- Acupuncture: results are conflicting.
- *Achillea wilhelmsii*: data flawed.
- *Adenia cissampeliodes*: not enough data available.
- Aromatherapy: not enough data available.
- Chinese herbal medicine: not enough data available.
- Garlic (*Allium sativum*): small effect but data not convincing.
- Ginseng (*Panax ginseng*): few studies available.
- Green coffee bean extract: not enough data available.
- Hawthorn (*Crataegus* spp): data contradictory and scarce.
- Hypnotherapy: may reduce blood pressure in the short-term yet not enough data available.
- Maritime pine (*Pinus pinaster*): may reduce antihypertensive requirements but not enough data available.
- Meditation: data contradictory and methodologically limited.
- Melatonin: small reduction in blood pressure but not enough data available.
- Pomegranate (*Punica granatum*): not enough data available.

- Probiotics: not enough data available.
- Reishi (*Ganoderma lucidum*): not enough data available.
- Sesame (*Sesamum indicum*) oil: not enough data available.
- Vitamin C: not enough data available.
- Vitamin E: not enough data available.

☻ *Unlikely to be beneficial*
- Breathing exercises: the device Resperate is unlikely to reduce blood pressure
- Ginkgo (*Ginkgo biloba*): no evidence of effectiveness
- Green algae (*Chlorella pyrenoidosa*): no evidence of effectiveness
- Homeopathy: no evidence of effectiveness
- Olive leaf (*Olea europea*): no evidence of effectiveness
- Red clover (*Trifolium subterraneum*): no evidence of effectiveness
- Soy: unlikely to reduce blood pressure

☒ *Likely to be ineffective or harmful*
- Chiropractic: data contradictory, benefit does not outweigh the risk

Table 5.2 Systematic up-to-date reviews of treatments that are beneficial or likely to be beneficial for hypertension

Treatment	Source	No. of trials/ patients	Original conclusion
Biofeedback	*Hypertens Res* 2003; **26**:37–46.	N=22/n=905	Biofeedback was more effective in reducing blood pressure in patients with essential hypertension than no intervention
Co-enzyme Q10	*J Hum Hypertens* 2007; **21**:297–306.	N=3/n=120	Coenzyme Q10 has the potential in hypertensive patients to lower systolic blood pressure by up to 17mm Hg and diastolic blood pressure by up to 10mm Hg without significant side effects
Fish oil	*Arch Intern Med* 1993; **153**: 1429–38.	N=17/n=not available	High doses of omega-3 fatty acids, generally more than 3g/day, can lead to relevant blood pressure reductions in individuals with untreated hypertension

Table 5.2 (Contd.)

Treatment	Source	No. of trials/ patients	Original conclusion
Qigong	*J Hypertension* 2007; **25**: 1525–32	N=12/n=1218	There is some encouraging evidence to suggest that qigong is effective for lowering systolic blood pressure. However, the conclusiveness of these findings is limited
Tai chi	*J Hypertension* 2007; **25**: 1974–5	N=5/n=298	For hypertension the evidence is encouraging, suggesting potential effectiveness. However, the number of trials and the total sample size are too small to draw any firm conclusions

Conclusions

- Biofeedback is beneficial for lowering blood pressure. Several other treatments are likely to be beneficial yet the evidence is not entirely convincing
- The risks of biofeedback are small
- The risk–benefit balance for biofeedback is positive
- Conventional treatments are almost certainly more effective than the above CAM options

Further reading

Richard CL, Jurgens TM. Effects of natural health products on blood pressure. *Ann Pharmacother* 2005; **39**:712–20.

Vora CK, Mansoor GA. Herbs and alternative therapies: relevance to hypertension and cardiovascular diseases. *Curr Hypertens Rep* 2005; **7**:275–80.

Biofeedback

What is it?
A method using instruments to perceive body functions in order to control those functions

How does it work?
Modifications of physiological process at will

How is it used?
Used by a range of different types of practitioners in order to control autonomic functions and generate a relaxation response

Are there any risks?
Some reports suggest biofeedback can cause or aggravate psychological problems such as anxiety

Peripheral arterial occlusive disease

Peripheral arterial occlusive disease

Profile

Peripheral arterial occlusive disease (PAOD) results from atherosclerosis distal to the arch of the aorta leading to impaired circulation to the extremities and other vital organs. Early symptoms include pain in the leg muscles, particularly calves, with walking or other vigorous exercise, which is relieved by pausing that activity (stage II PAOD, intermittent claudication). Severe aching pain in toes or feet at night and ulceration are signs and symptoms of more severe illness, which usually requires surgery. The major risk factors for PAOD include a history of smoking, diabetes, high blood pressure, high cholesterol levels, and age. Hydrotherapy, herbal medicine and lifestyle changes are frequently used for this condition.

Clinical bottom line

☺ Beneficial

- Ginkgo (*Ginkgo biloba*): increases in painfree and maximal walking distances in patients with intermittent claudication.
- Padma 28, a Tibetan herbal mixture: increases maximal walking distances in patients with intermittent claudication.

☻ Likely to be beneficial

- CO_2-applications: seem to improve pain-free walking distance.

☻ Unknown effectiveness

- Acupuncture: not enough data available for walking ability.
- Biofeedback: not enough data available for walking ability and pain.
- Garlic (*Allium sativum*): improvements in pain-free walking distance, not enough data available.
- Mediterranean diet: not enough data available.
- Vitamin E: insufficient evidence to determine its effectiveness.

☹ Unlikely to be beneficial

- Fish oil: unlikely to be beneficial.

✖ Likely to be ineffective or harmful

- Chelation therapy: likely to be ineffective and associated with considerable risks.

Table 5.3 Systematic, up-to-date reviews of treatments that are beneficial for peripheral arterial occlusive disease

Treatment	Source	No. of trials/patients	Original conclusion
Ginkgo	*Atherosclerosis* 2005; **181**:1–7	N=9/n=619	These results suggest that *Ginkgo biloba* extract is superior to placebo in the symptomatic treatment of intermittent claudication
Padma 28	*Atherosclerosis* 2006; **189**:39–46	N=5/n=272	Available evidence shows that Padma 28 provides significant relief from PAOD-related symptoms, probably of the same order of magnitude as other employed medications

Conclusions

- Data suggest effectiveness for ginkgo and Padma 28; CO_2-applications are likely to be beneficial
- Allergic reactions and herb–drug interactions are potentially serious risks. Gastrointestinal disturbances, pruritus, headache, dizziness, epi-leptic seizures should be considered as possible adverse events to gingko
- The risk–benefit balance for ginkgo and Padma 28 in patients with intermittent claudication is positive and likely to be positive for CO_2-applications
- Ginkgo seems to be as effective as other conventional oral drugs, but no therapy is as effective for intermittent claudication as regular physical exercise and smoking cessation

Further reading

White C. Clinical practice. Intermittent claudication. *N Engl J Med* 2007; **356**:1241–50.
Hankey GJ, Norman PE, Eikelboom JW. Medical treatment of peripheral arterial disease. *JAMA* 2006; **295**:547–53.

Ginkgo (Ginkgo biloba)

What is it?
A tree native to China, Korea, and Japan. Leaves are used for medicinal purposes

How does it work?
Increase of microcirculatory blood flow, inhibition of platelet and erythrocyte aggregation, platelet-activating factor antagonism, free radical scavenging

How is it used?
Orally, mostly as powdered extract

Are there any risks?
There is a possible risk of allergic reactions and drug interactions

Padma 28

What is it?
A Tibetan mixture of 20 herbal drugs, calcium, and camphor

How does it work?
Largely unknown, but antioxidative properties may play a prominent role

How is it used?
Orally

Are there any risks?
Mild and infrequent adverse events (e.g. gastrointestinal system disorders) are on record

Stroke

Profile

Stroke (also cerebrovascular accident) is defined as a focal or global loss of cerebral function usually due to cerebral haemorrhage or (more frequently) cerebral ischaemia (e.g. cerebral infarction caused by arteriosclerosis). The main risk factor is hypertension but other cardiovascular risk factors are also important. The symptoms occur suddenly and vary from minor neurological deficits to major, permanent damage or death. Many stroke patients try CAM during rehabilitation or to improve symptoms in cases of permanent deficits.

Clinical bottom line

😐 *Unknown effectiveness*

- Acupuncture: the evidence is not convincing as an aid for stroke rehabilitation.
- Aromatherapy: combined with acupressure it may reduce pain but data are weak.
- Biofeedback, electromyographic: whether it exerts a treatment benefit is unclear.
- Dan shen: may improve neurological deficit yet not enough data available for this Chinese herbal medicine.
- Fish oil: the evidence for stroke prevention is contradictory.
- Garlic (*Allium sativum*): lowers the risk of arteriosclerosis, whether it is effective for stroke prevention is, however, unclear.
- Ginkgo (*Ginkgo biloba*): preliminary data suggest positive effects after cerebral haemorrhage.
- Ginseng (*Panax notoginseng*): may improve symptoms and function but few data available.
- Imagery: preliminary data suggest better functional recovery.
- Meditation: may normalize hypertension, a major risk factor for stroke, whether it prevents stroke is, however, unclear.

🔯 *Likely to be ineffective or harmful*

- Calcium/vitamin D supplementation: ineffective for reducing the risk of cardiovascular events in healthy postmenopausal women.
- Folic acid supplementation: ineffective for reducing the risk cardiovascular disease and stroke.
- Homeopathy: arnica was shown to have no effect on stroke recovery
- Selenium: no effect on stroke prevention.

Conclusions

- No CAM therapy has been shown to convey significant benefit for stroke prevention, treatment or rehabilitation
- No serious risks have been reported for the above treatments but adverse events and interactions need to be considered
- The risk–benefit balance fails to be positive for any CAM treatment
- Conventional treatment seems more effective than any CAM options and should be employed

Further reading

Dobkin BH. Strategies for stroke rehabilitation. *Lancet Neurol* 2004; **3**:528–36.

Michael KM, Shaughnessy M. Stroke prevention and management in older adults. *J Cardiovasc Nurs* 2006; **21**(5, Suppl 1):S21–6.

Dermatology

Acne

Acne is a common inflammatory disorder of the sebaceous follicles of the skin. It is characterized by comedones, papules, pustules, inflamed nodules, superficial pus filled cysts, and (in extreme cases) canalizing and deep, inflamed, sometimes purulent sacs. Lesions are most common on the face, but the neck, chest, upper back, and shoulders may also be affected. Most common type is acne vulgaris, but approximately 20 sub-types are recognized. Herbal medicines are most commonly used to control infection, stop itching and improve symptoms.

Clinical bottom line

☺ *Likely to be beneficial*
- Zinc: oral and topical application.

☹ *Unknown effectiveness*
- Ayurvedic herbal medicine: best results for Sunder Vati for reducing lesions but not enough data available.
- Biofeedback-assisted relaxation and cognitive imagery: not enough data available.
- Traditional Chinese herbal medicine: different herbs tested.
- Gugulipid: comparable to tetracyclines but further trials are required.
- *Ocimum basilicum:* comparable to tetracyclines but not enough data available.
- *Ocimum gratissimum:* comparable to benzoyl peroxide but not enough data available.
- Tea tree (*Melaleuca alternifolia*): may be comparable to benzoyl peroxide and superior to placebo but not enough data available.
- Toto: studies are scarce and have methodological limitations.
- Yeast: *Saccharomyces cerevsisiae,* data are scarce.

Conclusions

- Encouraging results have been reported for oral and topical zinc, no convincing evidence exists for any other CAM treatments
- Zinc is considered relatively safe when taken at recommended doses
- The risk–benefit balance for zinc is positive
- The effect of zinc compared with conventional treatment is unclear

Further reading

Goodman G. Managing acne vulgaris effectively. *Aust Fam Physician* 2006; **35**:705–9.

Zaenglein AL, Thiboutot DM. Expert committee recommendations for acne management. *Pediatrics* 2006; **118**:1188–99.

Eczema

Profile

Eczema or atopic dermatitis is an inflammation of upper layer of the skin leading to persistent or recurring skin rashes. The signs include redness, oedema, crusting, flaking, blistering, cracking, oozing, and bleeding. The symptoms include itching, localized skin lesions. Related terms are atopic eczema or atopic dermatitis, contact dermatitis, xerotic eczema, and seborrheic dermatitis. Many eczema sufferers try CAM, particularly homeopathy, acupuncture or special diets.

Clinical bottom line

☺ Likely to be beneficial

- Probiotics: reduce symptoms in infants and children.
- Zemaphyte: a Chinese herbal mixture may reduce skin lesions but results are not entirely uniform.

☻ Unknown effectiveness

- Autogenic training: itching, long-term results are encouraging but not enough data available.
- Autologous blood therapy: not enough data available.
- Biofeedback: itching, severity of skin lesions, not enough data available.
- Black seed (*Nigella sativa*) oil: not enough data available.
- Borage (*Borago officinalis*) oil: conflicting results.
- German chamomile (*Matricaria recutita*): topical, not enough data available.
- Hypnotherapy: severity, not enough data available.
- Johrei healing: data are not convincing and scarce.
- Liquorice (*Glycyrrhiza glabra*): topical gel, not enough data available.
- Selenium: results contradictory.
- Shuangfujin (Chinese herbal medicine): not enough data available.
- St John's wort (*Hypericum perforatum*): topical, not enough data available.

✖ Likely to be ineffective or harmful

- Evening primrose (*Oenothera biennis*) oil: initial positive studies were superseded by more rigorous negative trials.
- Massage: no evidence for effectiveness.
- Zinc: no evidence of effectiveness.

Conclusions

- Probiotics and the Chinese herbal mixture Zemaphyte may be effective
- Only Zemaphyte is associated with serious risks
- For probiotics, the risk–benefit balance is likely to be positive
- Conventional treatments are probably more effective than CAM

Further reading

Artik S, Ruzicka T. Complementary therapy for atopic eczema and other allergic skin diseases. *Dermatol Ther* 2003; **16**:150–63.

Chronic venous insufficiency

Profile

Chronic venous insufficiency (CVI, synonymous post-thrombotic syndrome) is caused by poorly functioning valves within the veins. Blood flows through incompetent valves, causing blood in the legs to pool leading to persistent venous hypertension and varicosity of the superficial veins. CVI is more common among patients who are obese, pregnant, or who have a family history of the condition. Other causes include deep vein thrombosis and phlebitis. Symptoms include swelling, leg pain, itch, cramps, feeling of heaviness and distress about cosmetic appearance. Herbal medicine and hydrotherapy are popular complementary therapies.

Clinical bottom line

☺ *Beneficial*

- Horse chestnut (*Aesculus hippocastanum*): symptom relief and reductions of leg oedema.

☺ *Likely to be beneficial*

- Butcher's broom (*Ruscus aculeatus*): symptom relief and reductions in leg volume, ankle and leg circumferences with combination product Cyclo 3 fort.
- Gotu kola (*Centella asiatica*): symptom relief and reductions of leg oedema.
- Hydro-/balneotherapy: improvement of venous function.

☹ *Unknown effectiveness*

- Buckwheat (*Fagopyrum esculentum*): reduction in leg volume and symptom scores, not enough data available.
- French maritime pine (*Pinus pinaster*): not enough data available.
- Red vine leaf (*Vitis vinifera*): symptoms relief and reductions of leg circumferences, not enough data available.
- Vitamin E: symptom relief, not enough data available.

☒ *Likely to be ineffective or harmful*

- Ginkgo (*Ginkgo biloba*): likely to be ineffective.

Conclusions

- Best evidence supports the use of horse chestnut seed extract. A butcher's broom combination product, gotu kola and hydrotherapy are likely to be beneficial
- Allergic reactions to herbal medicines should be considered. Gastrointestinal discomfort and nausea may occur
- The risk–benefit balance is clearly positive for horse chestnut seed extract and likely to be positive for butcher's broom combination product, gotu kola, and hydrotherapy
- Compared to conventional treatments and suggestions that it may be as effective as compression therapy; horse chestnut seed extract is worthy of consideration

Further reading

Bergan JJ, Schmid-Schonbein GW, Smith PD et al. Chronic venous disease. *N Engl J Med* 2006; **355**:488–98.

Wollina U, Abdel-Naser MB, Mani R. A review of the microcirculation in skin in patients with chronic venous insufficiency: the problem and the evidence available for therapeutic options. *Int J Low Extrem Wounds* 2006; **5**:169–80.

Horse chestnut (*Aesculus hippocastanum*)

What is it?

A tree native to south-eastern Europe. The seeds are used medicinally

How does it work?

Antiexudative, anti-inflammatory, and immunomodulatory activity

How is it used?

Orally as standardized extract daily in divided doses and externally apply several times daily

Are there any risks?

Pruritus, nausea, gastrointestinal complaints, bleeding, dizziness, headache, nephropathy, allergic reactions, interactions

Hair loss

Profile

Hair loss (alopecia or baldness) can have many causes. The most common form is androgenic alopecia (male pattern baldness) which occurs in adult men and is thought to be due to genetic and hormonal factors. Men afflicted by this common (about 75% of all men over the age of 80) and gradually progressing condition are likely to try CAM, particularly topical and oral herbal medicines.

Clinical bottom line

😑 Unknown effectiveness

- Aromatherapy: preliminary data suggest positive effects in alopecia areata, not enough data available.
- Dabao (herbal extract): data are encouraging but preliminary.
- Garlic (*Allium sativum*), topical: as an adjunct to corticosteroids, not enough data available.
- Hypnotherapy: data are encouraging but preliminary.

😢 Unlikely to be beneficial

- Chinese herbal medicine: not effective for chemotherapy-associated hair loss.

Conclusions

- No CAM therapy is demonstrably effective
- No serious risks are associated with the above treatments
- A risk–benefit balance fails to be positive
- Androgenic alopecia is resistant to both conventional and CAM approaches. If alopecia is due to a specific cause, the elimination of that cause may restore hair growth

Further reading

Meidan VM, Touitou E. Treatments for androgenetic alopecia and alopecia areata: current options and future prospects. *Drugs* 2001; **61**:53–69.

Psoriasis

Profile

Psoriasis is a chronic inflammatory skin disease that is characterized by well demarcated erythematous scaly plaques on the extensor surfaces of the body and scalp. Chronic plaque psoriasis affects about 1–3% of the general population. It may also affect joints in about 10% and nails in up to one third of the cases. The condition affects both sexes equally and may appear at any age, although it is more likely between the ages of 11 and 45. About a third of psoriasis patients have a family history of the disease but the exact cause is not known.

Clinical bottom line

😊 Likely to be beneficial

- Capsaicin: seems to reduce itching, scaling, and erythema.
- Omega-3 fatty acids: may reduce severity when administered as infusions.

😐 Unknown effectiveness

- Aloe vera (*Aloe barbadensis*): few and conflicting data.
- Avocado oil: not enough data available.
- Homeopathy: independent replication for a *Mahonia aquifolium* product required.
- Hypnotherapy: not enough data available.

😟 Unlikely to be beneficial

- Acupuncture: not superior to placebo.
- Balneotherapy: no beneficial effects of saline water.
- Efamol (omega-3 fish oil and omega-6 evening primrose oil).
- Kukui nut oil: no difference to placebo.

Conclusions

- Capsaicin and omega-3 fatty acids are likely to be beneficial but the evidence is not entirely convincing
- Allergic reactions and vitamin D hypervitaminosis should be considered as adverse events to omega-3 fatty acids
- The risk–benefit balance for capsaicin and fish oil is likely to be positive
- Compared to conventional options, CAM treatments have only little to offer

Further reading

Smith CH, Barker JN. Psoriasis and its management. *BMJ* 2006; **333**:380–4.

Diabetology

Diabetes

Profile

Diabetes mellitus is a metabolic disorder affecting carbohydrate metabolism. It is characterized by hyperglycaemia, defined as a fasting plasma glucose ≥ 7.0mmol/L or ≥ 11.1mmol/L 2 hours after a 75g oral glucose load, on two or more occasions. Treatment aims to lower blood glucose levels to the non-diabetic range. The main approaches are education, monitoring, self management, and pharmacological treatment with insulin or oral anti-diabetic agents. Diabetes mellitus is a major risk factor for cardiovascular disease, chronic renal failure and neuronal damage. Herbal supplements are often used for this condition.

Clinical bottom line

☺ Beneficial

- Guar gum (*Cyamopsis tetragonolobus*): reduces total and LDL cholesterol levels in diabetic patients.
- Psyllium (*Plantago ovata*): reduces total and LDL cholesterol levels in diabetic patients.

☺ Likely to be beneficial

- Ayurveda: glucose lowering effects of *Coccinia indica* and *Gymnema sylvestre* deserving further study.
- Cinnamon (*Cinnamomum zeylanicum*): seems to reduce fasting blood glucose levels.
- Fish oil: may lower triglyceride levels in diabetic patients.
- Soy: beneficial effects for fasting insulin, insulin resistance and total and LDL levels in type 2 diabetes.

☹ Unknown effectiveness

- *Agaricus blazei murill*: a mushroom that may reduce insulin resistance
- Biofeedback: may decrease blood glucose and HbA1c but not enough data available.
- Blueberry leaf extract (*Vaccinum arctostaphylos*): may reduce plasma glucose yet not enough data available.
- Chinese herbal medicines: some beneficial effects reported but not convincing enough for any recommendations.
- Chromium: inconclusive data for glucose, insulin, HbA1c, and lipid levels.
- Co-enzyme Q10: not enough data available.
- Fenugreek (*Trigonella foenum-graecum*): some beneficial effects on blood glucose and triglyceride levels but not enough data available.
- French maritime pine (*Pinus pinaster*): may reduce blood glucose and slow the progression of diabetic retinopathy but not enough data available.
- Garlic (*Allium sativum*): may have small benefits on dyslipidaemia in diabetic patients.
- Ginseng (*Panax ginseng*): data are not convincing.

- Ginseng (*Panax quinquefolius*): some positive results exist but data are not convincing.
- Inolter: a herbal preparation that may lower blood glucose but not enough data available.
- *Ipomoea batatas*: some positive effects on glucose and cholesterol levels but not enough data available.
- Milk thistle (*Silybum marianum*): may reduce HbA1c, total and LDL cholesterol.
- Mulberry (*Morus indica*): may have hypoglycaemic and hypolipidaemic effects yet few data available.
- Pancreas tonic: a mixture of Indian Ayurvedic herbs that may improve glucose control but not enough data available.
- Qigong: insulin resistance in type 2 diabetes, not enough data available.
- Red clover (*Trifolium pratense*): blood pressure lowering effects in diabetic patients but not enough data available.
- Reflexology: not enough data available for glucose control.
- Taizhi'an: not enough data available for this traditional Chinese medicine (TCM).
- Tea (*Camellia sinensis*): not enough data available for oolong and green teas.
- Vitamin E: some beneficial effects are reported yet not enough data available.

😣 Unlikely to be beneficial
- Breathing exercises: seems to not reduce blood pressure or improve quality of life in diabetic patients.
- Jiangtang bushen recipe: seems to not reduce the risk of developing type 2 diabetes.

🗿 Likely to be ineffective or harmful
- Glucosamine: no effects on glycaemic control.
- Magnesium: no effects on glycaemic control.
- *Syzygium cumini*: no changes in fasting blood glucose levels.
- *Tinospora crispa*: no beneficial effects reported.
- Xioke tea: no beneficial effects reported.
- Zinc: no effects on HbA1c and glucose homeostasis.

Conclusions

- Best evidence suggests that guar gum and psyllium reduce total and LDL cholesterol levels in diabetic patients. Two Auyrvedic preparations, cinnamon, fish oil and soy are likely to have beneficial effects
- Fibre supplements should be taken with adequate amounts of fluid; allergic reactions should be considered
- The risk–benefit balance for guar gum and psyllium is positive and likely to be positive for the other above treatments
- Effective conventional options exist and CAM options, which only have modest effect sizes on metabolic control, should only be considered as adjuncts

Further reading

Daneman D. Type 1 diabetes. *Lancet* 2006; **367**:847–58.

Stumvoll M, Goldstein BJ, van Haeften TW. Type 2 diabetes: principles of pathogenesis and therapy. Lancet 2005; **365**:1333–46.

Guar gum

What is it?

Guar gum is derived from the Indian cluster bean (*Cyamopsis tetragonolobus* L.). Its main constituent is galactomannan.

How does it work?

Mainly by increasing the viscosity of the bowel content.

How is it used?

Orally, 9–15g daily.

Are there any risks?

Adverse effects reported include allergic reactions, flatulence, diarrhoea, abdominal pain and cramps. Drug interactions have been suggested.

Psyllium (Plantago ovata)

What is it?

An annual herb with bulk-forming laxative properties.

How does it work?

Decreases passage time through increases in stool volume.

How is it used?

Orally as dietary supplement.

Are there any risks?

Allergic reactions including anaphylaxis, possible interactions with cardiac glycosides.

Gastroenterology

Constipation

Profile

The Rome II criteria define chronic constipation (synonyms: obstipation, costiveness) on the basis of two or more of the following symptoms at least 25% of the time for at least 12 weeks in the preceding year: straining at defecation; stools that are lumpy/hard; sensation of incomplete evacuation; and three or fewer bowel movements a week. Herbal medicines are often used for this condition.

Clinical bottom line

☺ *Beneficial*

- Psyllium (*Plantago ovata*): evidence supports its use in chronic constipation.

☺ *Likely to be beneficial*

- Abdominal massage: may increase stool frequency and consistency but data scarce and methodologically limited.
- Biofeedback: seems to improve constipation and dyssynergic defecation.
- Fibre: may increase stool frequency in pregnancy-related constipation.

☻ *Unknown effectiveness*

- Acupuncture: may increase the frequency of bowel movement, not enough data available.
- *Aloe vera:* may increase the frequency of bowel movement, not enough data available.
- Ayurveda: not enough data available.
- Meditation: encouraging data available but replication required.
- Padma Lax: in constipation-predominant irritable bowel syndrome abdominal pain may decrease, not enough data available.
- Probiotics (*Lactobacillus casei*): improvement in severity of constipation and stool consistency, not enough data available.
- Herbal tea: a supplement (Smooth Move) showed increased bowel movements yet not enough data available.

☹ *Unlikely to be beneficial:*

- Probiotics (*Lactobacillus GG*): no improvement in spontaneous bowel movements.

☒ *Likely to be ineffective or harmful*

- Reflexology: no effects on stool frequency.

Table 5.4 Systematic up-to-date reviews of treatments that are beneficial or likely to be beneficial for constipation

Treatment	Source	No. of trials/ patients	Original conclusion
Biofeedback	*Dis Colon Rectum* 2003; **46**:1208–17	N=7/n=1081	Although most studies report positive results using biofeedback to treat constipation, quality research is lacking
Fibre	*Cochrane Database Syst Rev* 2001; **2**:CD001142	N=2/n=180	Dietary supplements of fibre in the form of bran or wheat fibre are likely to help women experiencing constipation in pregnancy
Psyllium (*Plantago ovata*)	*Am J Gastroenterol* 2005; **100**:936–71	N=7/n=856	There is good evidence to support the use of PEG, tegaserod, lactulose, and psyllium

Conclusions

- Best evidence supports the use of psyllium in chronic constipation. Fibre supplements in pregnancy-related constipation and constipation in irritable bowel syndrome patients, abdominal massage and biofeedback are likely to be beneficial
- For psyllium and fibre supplements allergic reactions should be considered. Other serious risks have not been reported. Fibre supplements should be taken with adequate amounts of fluid
- The risk–benefit balance for psyllium is positive and likely to be positive for fibre supplements, biofeedback and abdominal massage
- Compared to the risks of long-term conventional treatments, psyllium is a reasonable option for constipated patients

Further reading

DiPalma JA. Current treatment options for chronic constipation. Rev Gastroenterol Disord 2004; **4** (Suppl 2):S34–42.

Psyllium (*Plantago ovata*)

What is it?

An annual herb with bulk-forming laxative properties

How does it work?

Decreases passage time through increases in stool volume

How is it used?

Orally as dietary supplement

Are there any risks?

Allergic reactions including anaphylaxis, possible interactions with cardiac glycosides

Crohn's disease

Profile

Crohn's disease (synonym: Morbus Crohn) is an inflammation of the bowel of unknown origin. It can affect the gastrointestinal system anywhere from the mouth to the anus but most commonly affects the lower part of the small intestine. All layers of the intestine may be involved and healthy bowel can be found between sections of diseased bowel. It causes ulceration and swelling resulting in abdominal pain, often in the lower right area, and diarrhoea. Rectal bleeding, weight loss, arthritis, skin problems, and fever may also occur. Crohn's disease seems to run in families and can occur in people of all ages, though more commonly between the ages of 20 to 30. At present, there is no cure for Crohn's disease and treatment focuses on symptom relief. In severe cases, surgery may be necessary. Herbal and non-herbal dietary supplements as well as chiropractic, reflexology, and homeopathy are frequently used.

Clinical bottom line

😃 Likely to be beneficial
- Fish oil, omega-3 fatty acids: antiinflammatory effects.
- Probiotic (*Saccharomyces boulardii*): reduction in clinical relapses.

😐 Unknown effectiveness
- Acupuncture: decrease in disease activity but not enough data available.
- Biofeedback: not enough data available.
- Indian frankincense *(Boswellia serrata)*: decrease in disease activity with combination product but not enough data available.
- Relaxation: may reduce healthcare utilization but not enough data available.
- Vitamins: may be beneficial for correcting nutritional deficiencies.

😣 Unlikely to be beneficial
- Relaxation.

🗡 Likely to be ineffective or harmful
- Probiotic (*Lactobacillus GG*): likely to be ineffective.
- Probiotic (*Lactobacillus johnsonii LA1*): likely to be ineffective.

Conclusions

- *S. boulardii* preparations and fish oil are likely to be beneficial
- Serious risks may include rare allergic reactions to *S. boulardii*
- The risk–benefit balance fails to be clearly positive for any CAM treatment: fish oil and *S. boulardii* preparations however may be worth considering
- Compared with conventional therapy, CAM does not provide alternatives. Fish oil and *S. boulardii* should rather be considered as possible adjunctives

Further reading

Shanahan F. Crohn's disease. *Lancet* 2002; **359**:62–9.

Hepatitis

Profile

Inflammation of the liver normally caused by either viral infections (hepatitis A, B, C, D, E viruses) or toxic agents. The hepatitis B, C, and D viruses can cause chronic hepatitis, in which the infection is prolonged, sometimes lifelong. Symptoms include jaundice, fatigue, abdominal pain, loss of appetite and body weight, nausea, vomiting, diarrhoea, low grade fever, and headache. However, some people do not have symptoms and some chronic forms of hepatitis show very few of these signs. Several herbal medicines and some other food supplements are used. Others are implicated in causing toxic hepatitis.

Clinical bottom line

😊 *Likely to be beneficial*

- Milk thistle (*Silybum marianum*): encouraging results of silymarin for various forms of viral hepatitis, likely to decrease serum transaminases in patients with acute viral hepatitis.
- *Phyllanthus* spp: antiviral activity and liver biochemistry in chronic hepatitis B.
- Sho-saiko-to: a herbal mixture, improvement of liver enzymes, decrease of viral antigen.
- *Sophora flavescens*: the alkaloid matrine may have antiviral activity and positive effects on liver biochemistry in hepatitis B.

😐 *Unknown effectiveness*

- Ayurvedic herbal mixture: Kamalahar improves symptoms and liver enzymes but not enough data available.
- Chinese medicinal herbs: encouraging data exist for numerous Chinese herbs including *Astragalus polygonum*, Bin gan, Da Ding Feng Zhu, Fuzheng Huayu, Gaixan, Heije, Jiedu Yanggan Gao, Kangxian Baogan, Yi zhu, Yi er gan tan, Zhaoyangwan, yet data too few and in most cases methodologically weak.
- Enzyme therapy, oral: data are methodologically weak.
- Liquorice (*Glycyrrhiza glabra*): may improve virological or biochemical markers results are inconclusive.
- Sweet potato, purple (*Ipomoea batatas*): might affect serum hepatic biomarker levels in healthy adult men with borderline hepatitis but not enough data available.
- *Salvia miltiorrhiza/Polyporus umbellatus*: not enough data available.

😟 *Unlikely to be beneficial*

- Milk thistle (*Silybum marianum*): alcoholic and/or hepatitis B or C virus liver diseases.

☣ *Likely to be ineffective or harmful*

- Antioxidants: no effects on virological response.
- Liv 52O: Ayurvedic herbal mixture, increased mortality reported in one clinical trial.
- *Uncaria gambir*: burdened with significant toxicity.

Table 5.5 Systematic up-to-date reviews of treatments that are likely to be beneficial for hepatitis

Treatment	Source	No. of trials/ patients	Original conclusion
Milk thistle (*Silybum marianum*)	*J Viral Hepat* 2005; **12**:559–67	N=7/n=342	Silymarin compounds likely decrease serum transaminases in patients with acute viral hepatitis but do not seem to affect viral load or liver histology
Phyllantus spp	*J Viral Hepat* 2001; **8**:358–66	N=22/n=1947	Phyllanthus species may have positive effect on antiviral activity and liver biochemistry in chronic HBV infection
Sophora flavescens	*Am J Chin Med* 2003; **31**:337–54	N=22/n=2409	Sophorae flavescentis extract (matrine) may have antiviral activity and positive effects on liver biochemistry in chronic hepatitis B

Conclusions

- Encouraging effectiveness data exist for milk thistle, *Phyllanthus* spp, Sho-saiko-to, and *Sophora flavescens*
- No serious risks have been reported
- The risk–benefit balance for those herbal medicines is likely to be positive
- It is unclear how these treatments compare to conventional therapy such as interferon

Further reading

Coon JT, Ernst E. Complementary and alternative therapies in the treatment of chronic hepatitis C: a systematic review. *J Hepatol* 2004; **40**:491–500.

Irritable bowel syndrome

Profile

Irritable bowel syndrome (IBS) is a chronic non-inflammatory condition affecting the small and large bowel. It is a functional disorder with no apparent structural or biochemical abnormalities. The main symptoms are cramping, abdominal pain, altered bowel habit such as diarrhoea or constipation, and abdominal bloating. IBS affects approximately 15–20% of the general population and is one of the most common conditions seen by gastroenterologists and primary care physicians. It occurs more often in women than men and often between the ages of 25–45 years.

Clinical bottom line

😊 *Beneficial*

- Fibre supplementation: bulk forming agents seem beneficial for global symptom relief and IBS-related constipation.

😊 *Likely to be beneficial*

- Chinese herbs: seems to improve symptoms.
- Hypnotherapy: seems to improve symptoms and quality of life.
- Peppermint (*Mentha x piperita*): seems to improve symptoms.
- Probiotic (*Lactobacillus plantarum*): seems to be helpful for global improvement of symptoms.
- Psyllium (*Plantago ovata*): may be helpful for global improvement of symptoms.
- Tong Xie Yao Fang: may lead to symptom improvement.

😐 *Unknown effectiveness*

- Acupuncture: most trials are of poor quality.
- Biofeedback: as part of a multi-component treatment no effects on overall symptom scores.
- Carmint (*Melissa officinalis*, *Mentha spicata*, and *Coriandrum sativum*): may improve abdominal pain but not enough data available.
- Cognitive behaviour therapy: some positive effects but not enough data available.
- Florelax (yeast, vitamin B, nicotinamide, folic acid, herbal extracts of chamomile, angelica, valerian, peppermint): symptom improvement but only few data available.
- Iberogast (*Iberis amara*, *Chelidonii herba*, *Cardui mariae fructus*, *Melissae folium*, *Carvi fructus*, *Liquiritiae radix*, *Angelicae radix*, *Matricariae flos*, *Menthae piperitae folium*): may lead to symptom improvement including abdominal pain but too few data available.
- Meditation: few data and independent replication required.
- Padma Lax: a Tibetan herbal formula may improve symptoms yet only few data available.
- Probiotic (*Bifidobacterium infantis*, *Propionibacterium*, Prescript-Assist, VSL3): some positive effects reported yet not enough data available.
- Yoga: may improve symptoms but few data available.

😣 *Unlikely to be beneficial*
- Aloe vera (*Aloe barbadensis*): seems not effective but diarrhoea predominant patients showed a trend.
- *Asa foetida*: some benefits reported but not beyond placebo.
- Cognitive therapy: not better than attention placebo for symptom control.
- Probiotic (*Lactobacillus reuteri*, Medilac DS, *Bacillus subtilis*, *Streptococcus faecium*): no effects for symptom improvement and quality of life.
- Reflexology: seems not effective for improving abdominal pain, distension and constipation/diarrhoea.

🗶 *Likely to be ineffective or harmful*
- Appital: a herbal combination preparation, likely to be ineffective.
- Ayurveda: preparation containing *Aegle marmelos correa* and *Bacopa monnieri*, likely to be ineffective.
- *Curcuma xanthorriza*: likely to be ineffective for pain and distension.
- *Fumaria officinalis*: likely to be ineffective for pain and distension.

Table 5.6 Systematic up-to-date reviews of treatments that are likely to be beneficial for irritable bowel syndrome

Treatment	Source	No. of trials/patients	Original conclusion
Hypnotherapy	*Aliment Pharmacol Ther* 2006; **24**:769–80	N=18/n=926	The published evidence suggests that hypnotherapy is effective in the management of IBS.
Peppermint	*Phytomedicine* 2005; **12**:601–6	N=16/n=651	[...] administered orally in an enteric coated form is a safe, efficacious and cost-effective symptomatic short term treatment in reducing global symptoms and pain [...].
Tong Xie Yao Fang	*J Altern Complement Med* 2006; **12**:401–7	N=12/n=1125	There is evidence of potential usefulness of TXYF-A [Tong Xie Yao Fang with Chinese herbal medicines] for IBS patients.

Conclusions

- Best evidence suggests that fibre is beneficial for global symptom relief and IBS-related constipation. A number of other options are likely to be beneficial but the data are not fully convincing
- Fibre supplements should be taken with adequate amounts of fluid. Allergic reactions should be considered
- The risk–benefit balance for fibre is positive
- Many conventional options are also not fully convincing and it seems that some complementary treatments may be worth trying

Further reading

Hussain Z, Quigley EM. Systematic review: Complementary and alternative medicine in the irritable bowel syndrome. *Aliment Pharmacol Ther* 2006; **23**:465–71.
Talley NJ. Irritable bowel syndrome. *Intern Med J* 2006; **36**:724–8.

Fibre

What is it?

Dietary fibres are the indigestible portion of plant foods. Dietary fibre consists of polysaccharides and other plant components such as cellulose.

How does it work?

Insoluble fibre possesses water-attracting properties that increase bulk, soften stools, and shorten gastrointestinal transit time. Soluble fibre undergoes metabolic processing.

How is it used?

Orally, as supplements or with natural food intake.

Are there any risks?

Dietary fibre should be taken with adequate amounts of fluid, gastrointestinal obstruction is a contraindication.

Nausea and vomiting

Profile

Vomiting is the ejection of matter through the mouth from the stomach and nausea is the inclination to vomit or the sensation associated with vomiting. Nausea and vomiting associated with pregnancy, surgery, chemotherapy and motion will be considered. Acupuncture and acupressure are commonly used for nausea in early pregnancy, commercial acupressure wrist-bands for seasickness and various CAM methods may be used as adjuncts in cancer therapy. Ginger (*Zingiber officinale*) is a popular herbal remedy for nausea and vomiting.

Nausea of pregnancy

Clinical bottom line

☺ *Beneficial*

- Acupoint stimulation: finger or wristband acupressure and electrical acupoint stimulation reduce nausea and vomiting.

☯ *Trade off between benefits and harms*

- Ginger (*Zingiber officinale*): evidence of effectiveness but encouraging preliminary data on safety need to be confirmed in observational studies with larger sample size.

☹ *Unknown effectiveness*

- Acupuncture: data are conflicting.

Table 5.7 Systematic up-to-date reviews of treatments that are beneficial or likely to be beneficial for nausea and vomiting of pregnancy

Treatment	Source	No. of trials/patients	Original conclusion
Acustimulation (acupressure, acupuncture, electrostimulation)	*Explore (NY)* 2006; **2**:412–21	N=14/n=1655	Acustimulation reduced the proportion of nausea and vomiting […] Acupressure and electrical stimulation had greater impact than the acupuncture methods.
Ginger (*Zingiber officinale*)	*Obstet Gynecol* 2005; **105**:846–56.	N=7/n=862	Ginger may be an effective treatment for nausea and vomiting in pregnancy.

Conclusions

- Acupressure, electrical acupoint stimulation and ginger are effective treatments
- There are encouraging preliminary safety data for ginger but it remains contraindicated in pregnancy until these have been confirmed in larger trials; acupoint stimulation is only associated with minor adverse events
- The risk–benefit balance for acupoint stimulation is positive
- Considering the limited therapeutic options available during pregnancy, acupressure and electrical acupoint stimulation can be recommended, ginger should only be used with caution

Postoperative nausea and vomiting (PONV)

Clinical bottom line

:☺: *Beneficial*

- Acupoint stimulation: in adults acupuncture, acupressure, electrical stimulation, and acupoint stimulation with capsicum plaster reduced nausea, vomiting and use of rescue antiemetics: acupuncture is effective in reducing PONV in children.
- Ginger (*Zingiber officinale*): more effective than placebo in preventing PONV but effect probably of small clinical relevance.

☺ *Likely to be beneficial*

- Acupressure: may reduce symptoms in children but further data required.

☻ *Unknown effectiveness*

- Hypnotherapy: not enough data available.
- Peppermint (*Mentha piperita*) oil: not enough data available.

☹ *Unlikely to be beneficial*

- Electrical acupoint stimulation: no effect in reducing nausea in children.

✖ *Likely to be ineffective or harmful*

- Music therapy: no beneficial effects on PONV.

Table 5.8 Systematic up-to-date reviews of treatments that are beneficial or likely to be beneficial for postoperative nausea and vomiting

Treatment	Source	No. of trials/ patients	Original conclusion
Acupoint stimulation (adults)	*Explore (NY)* 2006; **2**:202–15	N=33/n=4204	Acupoint stimulation is just as effective as medications in reducing nausea and vomiting symptoms and acupressure is just as effective as acupuncture or electrical stimulation
Acupoint stimulation (children)	*Explore (NY)* 2006; **2**:314–20	N=12/n=1179	Acupressure and acupuncture are effective treatment modalities to reduce PONV in children
Ginger	*Am J Obstet Gynecol* 2006; **195**:95–9	N=5/n=363	This meta-analysis demonstrates that a fixed dose of at least 1g of ginger is more effective than placebo for the prevention of PONV

Conclusions

- There is evidence for acupoint stimulation techniques to reduce PONV in adults and children. Ginger has also been shown to be effective
- Acupoint stimulation is associated with mainly mild and minor risks, for ginger interactions must be considered
- The risk–benefit balance for acupoint stimulation and ginger (if interactions are avoided) is positive
- Benefits of acupoint stimulation in PONV are reported to be similar to those of antiemetic medication in both adults and children

Nausea and vomiting induced by chemotherapy
Clinical bottom line
😀 *Beneficial*
- Acupoint stimulation: adjunct stimulation with needles and electroacupuncture reduced the incidence of acute vomiting but not nausea, while acupressure reduced nausea but not vomiting.
- Relaxation: effective in preventing nausea and vomiting.

🙂 *Likely to be beneficial*
- Hypnotherapy: helpful for anticipatory and post-chemotherapy nausea in children and adolescents.

nditions

dyspepsia

to disorders of the stomach involving symptoms such
a, bloating, belching, or pain that can also develop in
al. Non-ulcer dyspepsia is a common, sometimes chro
upper gastrointestinal system, which may include
nach, and duodenum. Up to 20% of people suffer fr
st once a week. The exact cause of the condition is

m line

d caraway: combination preparations of Mentha x
arum carvi.

beneficial
hara scolymus): may relieve symptoms.

fectiveness
adjunctive treatment: not enough data available.
al medicine: not enough data available.
adjunctive treatment: only few data available.
ine (Hange-koboku-to): symptom improvement but
available.
Capsicum annuum): symptom improvement but too fe

rcuma longa): not enough data available.

ineffective or harmful
to be ineffective in Helicobacter pylori eradication.

te suggests that peppermint and caraway combination
s have effects of similar magnitude to conventional
Artichoke extract is likely to be beneficial
tions should be considered as adverse events but the
e for peppermint and caraway combination preparatior
ng
nefit balance for peppermint and caraway is positive an
positive for artichoke
o conventional options, peppermint and caraway
preparation is an option worth considering

ling
Deeks J et al. Pharmacological interventions for non-ulcer dyspepsia. Coch
v 2006; 4:CD001960.

☺ *Unknown effectiveness*
- Chinese herbal medicine: encouraging results for Huangqi but studies
  have methodological limitations.
- Massage: data conflicting.
- Music therapy: may have some effect but not enough data available.

☹ *Unlikely to be beneficial*
- Noninvasive electrostimulation.
- Guided imagery.

☒ *Likely to be ineffective or harmful*
- Biofeedback: not effective compared to relaxation therapy.

Conclusions

- Acupoint stimulation, relaxation and possibly hypnotherapy are
  effective adjuncts in chemotherapy-induced nausea and vomiting
- None of these therapies is associated with serious risks
- The risk–benefit balance for acupoint stimulation, relaxation and
  possibly hypnotherapy is positive
- None of these treatments were used instead of antiemetics

Table 5.9 Systematic up-to-date review of treatment that is beneficial
for nausea and vomiting induced by chemotherapy

Treatment	Source	No. of trials/ patients	Original conclusion
Acupoint stimulation	Cochrane Database Syst Rev 2006; 2:CD002285	N=11/n=1247	… suggesting a biologic effect of acupuncture point stimulation

Motion sickness
Clinical bottom line

☺ *Likely to be beneficial*
- Acupoint stimulation: experimentally induced motion sickness.

☺ *Unknown effectiveness*
- Ginger (Zingiber officinale): encouraging results but not enough data
  available.

☒ *Likely to be ineffective or harmful*
- Biofeedback: no effect compared with placebo feedback or no
  treatment.

Conclusions

- Acupoint stimulation might be effective
- It is not associated with serious risks
- The risk–benefit balance for acupoint stimulation in motion sickness
  is likely to be positive

Further reading

Streitberger K, Ezzo J, Schneider A. Acupuncture for nausea and vomiting: an update of clinical and experimental studies. *Auton Neurosci* 2006; **129**:107–17.
Jewell D, Young G. Interventions for nausea and vomiting in early pregnancy. *Cochrane Database Syst Rev* 2003; **4**:CD000145.

Acupuncture

What is it?

Treatment from TCM, usually with needle insertion at acupuncture points

How does it work?

In TCM, it is assumed that acupuncture restores the balance of yin and yang. Modern theories are based on neurophysiological concepts such as endorphin release or gate-control therapy

How is it used?

In TCM it is used as a panacea: in 'Western' acupuncture mainly for pain

Are there any risks?

Mild adverse effects occur in about 10% of patients, serious complications (e.g. pneumothorax) are rare

Ginger (*Zingiber officinale*)

What is it?

A perennial plant native to southern Asia

How does it work?

Antiemetic, anti-inflammmatory, positive inotropic, carminative, promotes secretion of saliva and gastric juices, cholagogue, inhibition of platelet aggregation

How is it used?

Orally as powdered extract

Are there any risks?

There is a theoretical risk of congenital deformity in neonates. Allergy to members of the *Zingiberaceae* family

Relaxation therapy

What is it?

Techniques for eliciting the nervous system

How does it work?

Progressive muscle relaxation in the normalizing of blood su consumption, heart rate, resp increases in skin resistance a techniques involve passive mus

How is it used?

Several months of daily practis the relaxation response

Are there any risks?

None known

Non-ulce

Profile

Dyspepsia refe
heartburn, nau
chest after a m
disorder of th
oesophagus, st
heartburn at le
known.

Clinical bot

Benefici

- Peppermint
  piperita and

Likely to b

- Artichoke (

Unknown

- Acupunctu
- Chinese he
- Homeopat
- Kampo me
  too few da
- Red peppe
  data availa
- Turmeric (

Likely to

- Fish oil: lik

Conclusio

- Best evid
  preparati
  medicatic
- Allergic r
  safety pre
  is encou
- The risk-
  likely to
- Compar
  combina

Further r

Moayyedi P, So
Database Sy

Caraway (*Carum carvi*)

What is it?
A biennial plant native to Europe and western Asia. Belongs to the carrot family (Apiaceae)

How does it work?
Antispasmodic, antimicrobial

How is it used?
Orally as extract in tablets or capsules

Are there any risks?
None known

Peppermint (*Mentha piperita*)

What is it?
A perennial herb, which grows throughout much of Europe and North America. A natural hybrid of water mint (*Mentha aquatica*) and spearmint (*Mentha spicata*)

How does it work?
Antispasmodic, antimicrobial, antiseptic, carminative, cholagogue, cooling. The principal active constituent of peppermint oil is thought to be menthol, a cyclic monoterpene with calcium channel-blocking activity

How is it used?
As infusion, dry extract, or essential oil daily in divided doses

Are there any risks?
Allergic reactions, skin irritation, contact dermatitis, laryngeal or bronchial spasm, heartburn. Contraindicated in children under the age of 12 years and in patients with obstruction of the bile duct

Ulcerative colitis

Profile

Ulcerative colitis, also named colitis ulcerosa, is an inflammatory bowel disease of unknown cause. It is characterized by periods of exacerbated symptoms predominately affecting the rectum and the colon. Inflammation and ulcers occur in the colon resulting in urgent and bloody diarrhoea, pain and continual tiredness. Ulcerative colitis is a rare disease, with an incidence of about 1 person per 10,000. The disease affects more women than men. Surgery with partial or total removal of the colon is occasionally necessary and can cure the disease.

Clinical bottom line

😃 Likely to be beneficial

- Fish oil: omega-3 fatty acids seems to reduce inflammation and thus steroid requirements.
- Probiotic (*Bifidobacteria*): seem to reduce disease activity index, prevent exacerbation, maintain remission.
- Probiotic (*Escherichia coli*): may maintain remission similar to mesalazine.
- Psyllium (*Plantago ovata*): seems to improve symptoms and maintain patients in remission.

😐 Unknown effectiveness

- Acupuncture: small reductions in disease activity but too few data available.
- Aloe vera (*Aloe barbadensis*): may reduce disease activity, too few data available.
- Biofeedback: very few data available.
- *Chlorella pyrenoidosa*: beneficial effects reported but too few data available.
- Curcumin: main constituent of *Curcuma longa* may reduce relapse frequency.
- Evening primrose (*Oenothera biennis*): may improve stool consistency but few data available.
- Folic acid: beneficial effects reported but too few data available.
- Jian Pi Ping: a Chinese herbal medicine for which few data exist.
- Kuijie powder: beneficial effects reported but too few data available.
- Probiotic (*Lactobacillus GG*): may increase relapse-free time yet not enough data available.
- Probiotic (VSL3): combination preparation for which few beneficial effects are reported.
- Relaxation: some data are reported in favour of progressive muscle relaxation but are not convincing.
- Wheat grass (*Triticum aestivum*): may reduce disease activity, too few data available.

Table 5.10 Systematic up-to-date review of treatment that is likely to be beneficial for ulcerative colitis

Treatment	Source	No. of trials/patients	Original conclusion
Fish oil	*Am J Clin Nutr* 2005; **82**:611–9	N=11/n=420	Data that pertain to the effects of n-3 fatty acids on steroid requirements suggest that n-3 fatty acids may reduce the need for or effective dose of corticosteroids among patients with IBD [ulcerative colitis]

Conclusions

- Best evidence suggests that there is no CAM intervention with convincing evidence of effectiveness. Fish oil, probiotic preparations of *E. coli* and *bifidobacteria* and psyllium are likely to be beneficial
- Allergic reactions, herb–drug interactions and vitamin D hypervitaminosis are adverse events that may occur with these interventions
- The risk–benefit balance for fish oil, probiotic preparations of *E. coli* and *bifidobacteria* and psyllium seems positive but is not entirely convincing
- Probiotics of *E. coli* and psyllium have been suggested to maintain remission to a similar extend as mesalazine but this is based on few data

Further reading

Kucharzik T, Maaser C, Lugering A et al. Recent understanding of IBD pathogenesis: implications for future therapies. *Inflamm Bowel Dis* 2006; **12**:1068–82.

Gynaecology and obstetrics

Labour

Profile

Labour (childbirth) is the act of giving birth to a baby. Labour pains are caused by rhythmical uterine contractions which under normal conditions increase in intensity, frequency, and duration, culminating in vaginal delivery of the infant. Hypnosis, acupuncture and some herbal medicines (particularly raspberry leaves) are commonly used therapies.

Clinical bottom line

:☺: *Beneficial*

- Hypnotherapy: reduces requirements for analgesics, fewer complications at birth.

☺ *Likely to be beneficial*

- Massage: pain relief, psychological support during labour.

☻ *Trade off between benefits and harms*

- Chanlibao: a Chinese herbal medicine preparation, might accelerate the second stage of labour compared with oxytocin but no comprehensive safety data available.
- Raspberry (*Rubus idaeus*) leaf: shortens second stage of labour but not enough data available: likely to be unsafe when concentrated raspberry leaf preparations are used during pregnancy because they may initiate labour, no systematic safety data available.

☻ *Unknown effectiveness*

- Acupuncture: encouraging evidence as an adjunct to conventional pain control but data are scarce and contradictory: insufficient evidence available for acupuncture for inducing labour.
- Aromatherapy: very little data available for pain relief which also have methodological limitations.
- Biofeedback: data for pain relief are conflicting.
- Transcutaneous electrical nerve stimulation (TENS): not enough data available for pain relief.

☻ *Unlikely to be beneficial*

- Music: no effects on pain.
- Reflexology: onset or duration of labour.

☒ *Likely to be ineffective or harmful*

- Homeopathy: no effects on cervical ripening or induction of labour.

Table 5.11 Systematic up-to-date review of treatment that is beneficial for labour

Treatment	Source	No. of trials/ patients	Original conclusion
Hypnotherapy	*Br J Anaesth* 2004; **93**:505–11	N=6/n=784	The evidence presented suggests that hypnosis, alone or in combination with other anaesthetic techniques, may offer advantages over conventional analgesia alone

Conclusions

- The evidence of effectiveness for the reduction of labour pain is positive for hypnotherapy and encouraging for massage
- No serious risks are associated with these treatments
- The risk–benefit balance for hypnotherapy is positive and for massage likely to be positive
- No CAM treatment is superior to conventional treatment but may be more acceptable to some women due to the concerns surrounding the effects of pharmacological anaesthesia on progress of labour and the neonate

Further reading

Smith C, Collins C, Cyna A, Crowther C. Complementary and alternative therapies for pain management in labour. *Cochrane Database Syst Rev* 2006; **4**:CD003521.

Hypnotherapy

What is it?

The induction of a trance-like state to facilitate relaxation and make use of enhanced suggestibility to treat psychological and medical conditions and affect behavioural changes.

How does it work?

Induction of the hypnotic trance where the patient's focus of attention is directed inwards, thereby allowing easier access to the non-critical unconscious mind which is more receptive to suggestion. Hypnosis is usually associated with a deep state of relaxation.

How is it used?

Varies according to the individual, but an average course is 6–12 weekly sessions.

Are there any risks?

Recovering repressed memories can be painful and psychological problems may be exacerbated. Psychosis and personality disorders are contraindicated.

Menopause

Profile

The physiological end of regular menstruations is often accompanied by mood changes, hot flushes, night sweats, insomnia, vaginal dryness, decreased libido, impairment of cognitive function, and other symptoms. The exact cause of most of these complaints is still not completely understood. Concerns about hormone replacement therapy have recently emerged and many women are keen to try CAM for controlling these troublesome symptoms. Herbal supplements and homeopathy seem particularly popular.

Clinical bottom line

☻ *Likely to be beneficial*

- Ginkgo (*Ginkgo biloba*): data suggest that it improves cognitive function in menopausal women.
- Red clover (*Trifolium pratense)*: seems to reduce the frequency of hot flushes.
- St John's wort (*Hypericum perforatum*): seems to improve mild-to-moderate depression.
- Relaxation: preliminary data imply positive effects on hot flushes but it is unclear which type of relaxation is best.

⊕ *Trade off between benefits and harms*

- Black cohosh (*Actaea racemosa*): seems to reduce depression and improve sleep quality but data on vasomotor symptoms are contradictory and it has been associated with liver damage.
- Kava (*Piper methysticum*): seems to reduce anxiety but has been associated with liver damage.

☹ *Unknown effectiveness*

- Acupuncture: results are contradictory for symptom control.
- Fennel (*Foeniculum vulgare*), a pollen extract: reduces hot flushes according to preliminary data.
- Osteopathy: not enough data available for hot flushes.
- Soy/phytoestrogens: data are highly contradictory for symptom improvement.
- Vitamin E: data are contradictory.

☹ *Unlikely to be beneficial*

- Ginseng (*Panax ginseng*): no improvement of quality of life, hot flushes or vaginal cytology.
- Ginkgo (*Ginkgo biloba*): no effect on menopause-associated depression.

✖ *Likely to be ineffective or harmful*

- Dong quai (*Angelica sinensis*): no evidence of effectiveness.
- Evening primrose (*Oenothera biennis*) oil: no evidence of effectiveness for bone density, hot flushes.
- Kudzu (*Pueraria lobata*): no evidence of effectiveness.
- Wild yam (*Dioscorea villosa*): no evidence of effectiveness.

Table 5.12 Systematic up-to-date review of treatment that is likely to be beneficial for menopausal symptoms

Treatment	Source	No. of trials/ patients	Original conclusion
Red clover	*Phytomedicine* 2007; **14**:153–9	N=11/n=1160	There is evidence of a marginally significant effect of *T. pratense* isoflavones for treating hot flushes in menopausal women

Conclusions

- Ginkgo, red clover, St John's wort, relaxation, black cohosh and kava may be effective in relieving menopause-associated symptoms such as hot flushes and depression
- Black cohosh and kava have been associated with liver damage; interactions of St John's wort need to be considered; none of the other above treatments are burdened with serious risks
- The risk–benefit balance for ginkgo, red clover, St John's wort, and relaxation is likely to be positive
- Conventional hormone replacement therapy is supported by stronger evidence than CAM for controlling menopausal symptoms

Further reading

Carroll DG. Nonhormonal therapies for hot flashes in menopause. *Am Fam Physician* 2006; **73**:457–64.

Nedrow A, Miller J, Walker M et al. Complementary and alternative therapies for the management of menopause-related symptoms: a systematic evidence review. *Arch Intern Med* 2006; **166**:1453–65.

Premenstrual syndrome

Profile

Premenstrual syndrome is a common set of symptoms which occurs during the late luteal phase of the menstrual cycle just before the onset of menstruation and resolves at the end of menstruation. Other terms are late luteal phase or premenstrual dysphoric disorder and premenstrual tension. The vast majority of menstruating women (about 95%) are affected by it but debilitating illness is much rarer (about 5%). Symptoms include nervous tension, depressive or aggressive mood swings, pelvic pain and nostalgia. Affected women and their families often suffer severely from these regular problems. Most women would therefore consider trying CAM, in particular dietary supplements.

Clinical bottom line

☹ *Unknown effectiveness*

- Acupuncture: some trials suggest that it alleviates dysmenorrhoea but methodological flaws prevent firm conclusions.
- Biofeedback: may reduce psychological and affective symptoms but not enough data available.
- Chaste tree (*Vitex agnus-castus*): results contradictory.
- Chiropractic: symptom control, too few studies available.
- Ginkgo (*Ginkgo biloba*): preliminary data for breast pain and nostalgia but more data required.
- Homeopathy: not enough data available.
- Massage: not enough data available.
- Meditation: trial data are encouraging but methodologically weak.
- Reflexology: preliminary results positive but confirmation is needed.
- Relaxation: not enough data available.
- Soy isoflavones: not enough data available.

☹ *Unlikely to be beneficial*

- Evening primrose (*Oenothera biennis*) oil: the best evidence fails to show effectiveness for symptom control including mastalgia.

Conclusions

- No CAM approach has been convincingly shown to reduce the symptoms of premenstrual syndrome
- Most of the treatments in question are not burdened with serious risks
- A risk–benefit analysis is not positive
- Reasonable good evidence exist for exercise, vitamin B$_6$, calcium or magnesium supplements which are not considered to be CAM

Further reading

Kronenberg F, Fugh-Berman A. Complementary and alternative medicine for menopausal symptoms: a review of randomized, controlled trials. *Ann Intern Med* 2002; **137**:805–13.

Rapkin A. A review of treatment of premenstrual syndrome and premenstrual dysphoric disorder. *Psychoneuroendocrinology* 2003; **28**(3):39–53.

Infectious diseases

AIDS/HIV infection

Profile

Following an infection with a human immunodeficiency virus (HIV) there is typically a period of 8–10 years during which the patient is HIV-positive yet free of symptoms. This is followed by a period of increasingly severe symptoms, the nature of which are highly variable. This stage of the infection is called acquired immune deficiency syndrome (AIDS). About 40 million people are infected with HIV worldwide. Unprotected sex is the most important risk factor. Most symptomatic patients will try some form of CAM including herbal medicines or other dietary supplements, acupuncture, massage, or meditation. Most CAM approaches that are beneficial or possibly beneficial are for palliative or supportive care rather than for curative therapy.

Clinical bottom line

☼ Beneficial

- Stress management: effective for reducing anxiety and anger or improve self-esteem, wellbeing, or quality of life.

☺ Likely to be beneficial

- Massage: may improve quality of life and possibly stimulate the immune system.
- Multivitamin: HIV-positive breastfeeding mothers may reduce HIV transmission rates through multivitamin supplementation.

☹ Unknown effectiveness

- Boxwood (*Buxus sempervirens*): not enough data available.
- Guided imagery: not enough data available.
- Homeopathy: not enough data available.
- Meditation: for stress, anxiety or anger, not enough data available.
- Selenium: not enough data available.
- Spiritual healing: for reduction of anxiety, not enough data available.
- Tai chi: for tension and anxiety, not enough data available.
- Tea tree oil (*Melaleuca alternifolia*): for oral candidiasis, not enough data available.
- Yogic breathing: for stress reduction, not enough data available.

☹ Unlikely to be beneficial

- Acupuncture: for neuropathic pain studies were negative.
- Chinese herbal mixture: many different preparations exist, data not encouraging.
- Distant healing: did not improve selected clinical outcomes.

✖ Likely to be ineffective or harmful

- Capsaicin: (topical) for pain, no evidence of effectiveness.
- Ozone therapy: to boost immunological defence, no evidence of effectiveness.

- Probiotics: for diarrhoea, no evidence of effectiveness.
- St John's wort (*Hypericum perforatum*): for antiviral activity, no evidence of effectiveness.

Conclusions

- Stress management has a role in supportive care. Massage may improve quality of life and multivitamins may be advisable for breastfeeding HIV-positive mothers
- None of these approaches is associated with serious risks
- The risk–benefit balance for all these treatments is therefore positive or likely to be positive
- These CAM approaches are mere adjuncts to conventional care and do not compete with mainstream therapies

Further reading

Liu JP, Manheimer E, Yang M. Herbal medicines for treating HIV infection and AIDS. *Cochrane Database Syst Rev* 2005; **3**:CD003937.

Mills E, Wu P, Ernst E. Complementary therapies for the treatment of HIV: in search of the evidence. *Int J STD AIDS* 2005; **16**:395–403.

Stress management

What is it?

Stress management comprises techniques intended to equip a person with effective coping mechanisms for dealing with psychological stress. Stress is hereby defined as a person's physiological response to an internal or external stimulus that triggers the fight-or-flight response

How does it work?

Depending on the theoretical paradigm, techniques of stress management are usually aimed at providing strategies to help individuals to cope with stressors or to understand the nature of their thought. Techniques may include autogenic training, cognitive therapy, conflict resolution, exercise, meditation, and progressive relaxation

How is it used?

Depending on the techniques used, they are initially taught in group or individual sessions with an aim of the individual being able to practice the techniques individually

Are there any risks?

None known

Athlete's foot

Profile

Athlete's foot or tinea pedis is a fungal infection of the skin of the foot, usually between the toes, caused by parasitic fungi. It causes scaling, flaking, and itching of the affected skin. Blisters and cracked skin may also occur, leading to exposed raw tissue, pain, swelling, and inflammation. The infection can be spread to other areas of the body, such as the armpits, knees, and elbows. Growth of the fungi is promoted by a dark, warm, moist environment such as that found inside shoes. The fungi persist for a long time in the environment, facilitating transmission of the disease in communal areas. Complementary treatment approaches include herbal medicine and urine therapy.

Clinical bottom line

☻ *Unknown effectiveness*

- *Acalapha wilkesiana*: may improve cure rate but data methodologically weak.
- Bitter orange (*Citrus aurantium*): may improve cure rate yet data are scarce methodologically weak.
- *Solanum chrysotrichum*: may improve signs and symptoms yet data scarce.
- Tea tree (*Melaleuca alternifolia*) oil: data contradictory.

Conclusions

- Best evidence fails to suggest that any CAM is of proven effectiveness for athlete's foot as a primary or adjunctive treatment
- The tested medicines seem relatively safe
- The risk–benefit balance fails to be positive for any CAM
- There are effective conventional options and CAM has little to offer for patients with athlete's foot

Further reading

Crawford F, Hart R, Bell-Syer SE *et al.* Extracts from "Clinical evidence": Athlete's foot and fungally infected toenails. *BMJ* 2001; **322**:288–9.

Diarrhoea

Profile

Diarrhoea is watery or liquid stools, usually with an increase in stool weight above 200g daily and an increase in daily stool frequency. In the UK an incidence of 19 cases per 100 person years has been reported, of which 3.3 cases per 100 person years resulted in consultation with a GP. The cause of diarrhoea depends on geographical location, standards of food hygiene, sanitation, water supply, and season. Commonly identified causes of sporadic diarrhoea in adults in developed countries include *Campylobacter*, *Salmonella*, *Shigella*, and *Escherichia coli*. In developed countries, death from infectious diarrhoea is rare, although serious complications, including severe dehydration and renal failure, can occur and may necessitate admission to hospital. Elderly people, infants and those in long-term care have an increased risk of death. CAM treatments often used are probiotics.

Clinical bottom line

☺ *Beneficial*

- Probiotics, prevention: beneficial for preventing acute diarrhoea of diverse causes in children and adults.

☺ *Likely to be beneficial*

- Probiotics, treatment: appears to be a useful adjunct to rehydration therapy in acute infectious diarrhoea in adults and children.

☻ *Unknown effectiveness*

- Carob bean juice: may reduce duration and stool output yet too few data available.
- Dowdo: a wheat-milk gruel that may improve frequency and duration of diarrhoea but published data contradictory.
- Guar gum (*Cyamopsis tetragonolobus*): may reduce duration of diarrhoea but not enough data available.
- Homeopathy: may be beneficial for childhood diarrhoea yet too few data available.
- Psyllium (Isphagula, *Plantago ovata*): may improve urgency and stool consistency but more data required.

Table 5.13 Systematic up-to-date review of treatment that is beneficial for diarrhoea

Treatment	Source	No. of trials/ patients	Original conclusion
Probiotics (prevention)	*Lancet Infect Dis* 2006; **6**:374–82	N=34/4844	... sufficient evidence for the role of probiotics in the prevention of acute diarrhoea. Although higher in children, the effect of probiotics is also observed in adults

Conclusions

- Best evidence suggests that probiotics are beneficial for preventing acute diarrhoea of diverse causes in children and adults. Probiotics are also likely to be beneficial for treating acute infectious diarrhoea
- There are no serious adverse events on record for probiotics
- The risk–benefit balance of probiotics is positive for preventing and likely to be positive for treating acute diarrhoea of diverse causes in children and adults

Further reading

Al-Abri SS, Beeching NJ, Nye FJ. Traveller's diarrhoea. *Lancet Infect Dis* 2005; **5**:349–60.
Starr J. *Clostridium difficile* associated diarrhoea: diagnosis and treatment. *BMJ* 2005; **331**:498–501.

Probiotics

What is it?

Probiotics are dietary supplements containing potentially beneficial bacteria or yeast.

How does it work?

Intended to assist the body's naturally occurring gut flora to re-establish itself after for instance antibiotic therapy.

How is it used?

Orally in dairy products and as tablets or capsules.

Are there any risks?

Some adverse events such as diarrhoea, bloating, flatulence and constipation have been reported.

Herpes simplex

Profile

A variety of conditions (cold sores, herpes labialis, herpes genitalis) caused by infection with herpes simplex virus types 1 and 2 marked by painful, watery blisters in most commonly the skin or mucous membranes or on the genitals. Herbal creams for the treatment of acute lesions or the prevention of recurrences are popular.

Clinical bottom line

☹ *Unknown effectiveness*

- Lemon balm (*Melissa officinalis*): herpes labialis treatment but not enough data available.
- Propolis: faster healing time and reduced incidence of superinfection than with placebo or acyclovir in genital herpes but not enough data available.
- Rhubarb (*Rheum palmatum*) and sage (*Salvia officinalis*) combination: as effective as aclovir in the treatment of herpes labialis but not enough data available.
- Shenqi: Chinese herb, reduced recurrence rate of genital herpes but only few data available.
- Siberian ginseng (*Eleutherococcus senticosus*): improvements in severity, duration and frequency of attacks but not enough data available.

☹ *Unlikely to be beneficial or harmful*

- Echinacea purpurea extract: no benefit in genital herpes.
- Tea tree (*Melaleuca alternifolia*): not effective in the treatment of recurrent herpes labialis.
- Vitamin A: no decrease in herpes simplex virus shedding and infectivity in genital herpes.

Conclusions

- There is no compelling evidence for any form of CAM in the treatment of herpes simplex
- None of the treatments is associated with serious risks but adverse events and interactions need to be considered
- The risk–benefit balance fails to be positive for any CAM treatment

Further reading

Perfect MM, Bourne N, Ebel C, Rosenthal SL. Use of complementary and alternative medicine for the treatment of genital herpes. *Herpes* 2005; **12**:38–41.

Herpes zoster

Profile

Herpes zoster (also: shingles, postherpetic neuralgia) is caused by activation of latent varicella-zoster virus (human herpes virus 3) in people who have been rendered partially immune by a previous attack of chickenpox. It infects the sensory ganglia and their areas of innervation and is characterized by pain along the distribution of the affected nerve, as well as crops of clustered vesicles over the area. CAM therapies are used to either relieve postherpetic pain symptoms or to enhance the healing process of the infection. Acupucuncture is advocated during both infection and to treat neuralgia.

Clinical bottom line

🙁 *Unknown effectiveness*

- Acupuncture: data conflicts whether or not acupuncture reduces post-herpetic pain.
- Capsaicin: pain reduction but effects are small.
- TCM: combination of Chinese medicine and mecobalamin superior at relieving pain than both on their own but not enough data available.
- *Clinacanthus nutans*: faster healing of skin lesions but data scarce.
- Geranium (*Pelargonium* spp) oil: pain reduction but not enough data available.
- Tai chi: increase in varicella-zoster specific cell-mediated immunity but not enough data available.

Conclusions

- There is no compelling evidence of effectiveness for any CAM treatment
- No serious risks have been reported for the above treatments
- The risk–benefit balance fails to be positive for any CAM treatment

Further reading

Dworkin RH, Johnson RW, Breuer J et al. Recommendations for the management of herpes zoster. *Clin Infect Dis* 2007; **44**(1):S1–26.

Malaria

Profile

Malaria is the most serious parasitic disease known to mankind. It is caused by protozoan infection of the red blood cells with one or more of the four species of the genus *Plasmodium*. Symptoms vary greatly and include spiking fevers, headache, muscular pain and weakness, convulsions, vomiting, cough, diarrhoea and abdominal pain. Organ failure, circulatory collapse, coma and death may ensue. About 5% of the world's population are affected, and malaria is endemic in more than 100 countries. The annual death rate exceeds 125 million. Preventative measures are of prime importance.

Clinical bottom line

☻ *Unknown effectiveness*

- Acupuncture has been suggested as an add-on to conventional therapy but the evidence is not convincing.

☒ *Likely to be ineffective or harmful*

- Homeopathy: homeopaths often recommend 'homeopathic vaccination' for malaria however there is no evidence that this approach is effective.

Conclusions

- Artemisinin originates from a plant used in TCM but, as a single chemical entity, it must be considered a conventional treatment
- No CAM therapy has been shown effective for malaria
- The risk–benefit balance for CAM fails to be positive
- Compared to conventional treatments CAM has little to offer to malaria patients

Further reading

Ashley E, McGready R, Proux S, Nosten F. Malaria. *Travel Med Infect Dis* 2006; **4**:159–73.

Metabolism/endocrinology

Hypercholesterolaemia

Profile

Hypercholesterolaemia—high levels of cholesterol in the blood—is a risk factor for atherosclerosis. Possible findings are yellowish patches around the eyelids (xanthelasma palpabrum) and white discoloration of the peripheral cornea (arcus senilis). Lowering the intake of saturated fats, in particular, will lower cholesterol levels and reduce the risk of atherosclerosis.

Clinical bottom line

☺ *Beneficial*

- Guar gum (*Cyamopsis tetragonolobus*): shown to lower total and LDL cholesterol levels.
- Oat: as well as other fibre products it has been shown to modestly reduce total and LDL cholesterol.
- Soy: reduces total cholesterol and LDL.

☺ *Likely to be beneficial*

- Artichoke (*Cynara scolymus*): some positive data, but evidence is not compelling.
- Chitosan: may reduce total and LDL cholesterol.
- Fish oil (omega-3 fatty acids): reductions in triglyceride levels and increases HDL levels.
- Psyllium (*Plantago ovata*): may modestly reduce total and LDL cholesterol.
- Red yeast rice: may reduce total, LDL cholesterol and triglyceride levels yet quality of data uncertain.
- Yoga: may reduce total cholesterol.

☺ *Unknown effectiveness*

- Dai-saiko-to: not enough data available.
- Fenugreek (*Trigonella foenum-graecum*): may reduce total cholesterol, HDL, and LDL cholesterol but not enough data available.
- Green tea (*Camellia sinensis*): reductions of total and LDL cholesterol reported but not enough data available.
- Guggul (*Commiphora mukul*): reductions of total cholesterol reported but data are contradictory.
- Konjac glucomannan: reductions of total and LDL cholesterol reported but not enough data available.
- Ozone therapy: few data available.
- Probiotic (*Bifidobacterium longum* BL1): reductions of total cholesterol reported but not enough data available.
- Vitamin E: few data available.

😣 *Unlikely to be beneficial*
- Co-enzyme Q10: no reductions of total cholesterol reported.
- Garlic (*Allium sativum*): may cause a small reduction of total cholesterol but effect is too small to be clinically meaningful.
- Ginseng (*Panax ginseng*): no difference to placebo reported for cholesterol levels.
- Saiko-ka-ryukotsu-borei-to: no relevant changes in total cholesterol.

🔯 *Likely to be ineffective or harmful*
- Aloe vera (*Aloe barbadensis*): no effects on LDL, HDL and total cholesterol.
- Seal oil: no effects on HDL and total cholesterol.

Table 5.14 Systematic up-to-date reviews of treatments that are beneficial or likely to be beneficial for hypercholesterolaemia

Treatment	Source	No. of trials/ Patients	Original conclusion
Red yeast rice	*Chin Med* 2006; 1:4	N=93/n=9625	Current evidence shows short-term beneficial effects of red yeast rice preparations on lipid modification
Soy isoflavones	*Am J Clin Nutr* 2007; 85:1148–56	N=11/n=780	Soy isoflavones significantly reduced serum total and LDL cholesterol but did not change HDL cholesterol and triacylglycerol

Conclusions

- Guar gum, oat, and soy are beneficial for hypercholesterolaemia. A number of other interventions are likely to be beneficial but the evidence is not entirely convincing
- Allergic reactions and drug interactions should be considered. Adverse events may include flatulence, diarrhoea, nausea, and hypoglycaemic symptoms. Guar gum should be taken with adequate amounts of fluid. Soy may affect the menstrual cycle
- The risk–benefit balance for guar gum, oat, and soy is positive and likely to be positive for several other interventions
- Compared with conventional options the effect sizes that can be achieved with CAM are moderate

Further reading

Crouse JR 3rd, Elam MB, Robinson JG et al. Cholesterol management: targeting a lower LDL cholesterol concentration increases adult treatment panel-III goal attainment. *Am J Cardiol* 2006; **97**:1667–9.

Guar gum

What is it?
Guar gum is derived from the Indian cluster bean (Cyamopsis tetra-gonolobus L.). Its main constituent is galactomannan.

How does it work?
Mainly by increasing the viscosity of the bowel content.

How is it used?
Orally, 9–15g daily.

Are there any risks?
Adverse effects reported include allergic reactions, flatulence, diarrhoea, abdominal pain and cramps. Drug interactions have been suggested.

Oat (Avena sativa)

What is it?
The oat is a species of cereal grain and grown throughout the temperate zones

How does it work?
Soluble fibre from oat bran is believed to lower cholesterol levels, and possibly reduce the risk of heart disease

How is it used?
Orally as food or dietary supplement

Are there any risks?
None

Soy

What is it?
Subtropical plant native to southeastern Asia

How does it work?
Components of soy, called isoflavones, are thought to have estrogen like effects on the body

How is it used?
Soy can be taken in a range of ways from isolated soy proteins to tea or milk

Are there any risks?
Allergic reactions have been reported

Overweight/obesity

Profile

Obesity is a chronic condition characterized by an excess of body fat to an extent that it poses a risk factor for certain conditions. Excessive body weight has been shown to predispose to cardiovascular diseases, diabetes mellitus type 2, osteoarthritis, some cancers, and other conditions. Adults with a body mass index (BMI) between 25–30 kg/m^2 are categorized as overweight, and those with a BMI above 30 kg/m^2 are categorized as obese. In the UK, an estimated 23% of men and 25% of women can be classified as obese amounting to a serious public health problem. Large numbers of CAM interventions are promoted for reducing body weight, but few have been rigorously tested.

Clinical bottom line

Diet and exercise are not viewed as complementary within the context of this assessment.

😊 Likely to be beneficial

- *Garcinica cambogia*: encouraging but too few data for reducing body weight.
- Hypnotherapy: may lead to small reductions in body weight.

😐 Trade off between benefits and harms

- *Ephedra sinica*: promotes modest weight loss but is associated with considerable adverse effects including cardiovascular risks.

😕 Unknown effectiveness

- Acupressure: may be helpful in weight loss maintenance but data not convincing.
- Acupuncture: no convincing evidence, data contradictory.
- Ayurveda: not enough data available.
- Capsaicin: may reduce body fat mass but not enough data available.
- *Cissus quadrangularis*: some positive effects reported but too few data available.
- Conjugated linoleic acid: may reduce body fat mass.
- Glucomannan: encouraging but few data on weight loss.
- Grape seed: not enough data available.
- Green tea (*Camellia sinensis*): data contradictory.
- Homeopathy: not enough data available.
- *Magnolia officinalis/Phellondendron amurense*: combination preparation reported to have some effects but too few data available.
- *Phaselus vulgaris:* not enough data available.
- Soy: not enough data available.
- Yohimbine: data are conflicting with regards to reduction of body weight.

😣 Unlikely to be beneficial

- Capsaicin: no effect on weight regain after reducing weight.
- Chitosan: high quality trials indicate minimal effects.
- Chromium: only minimal, if any, effects.
- *Citrus aurantium*: no benefit for reducing weight.

- Garlic (*Allium sativum*): no effect on lipid profile in overweight patients with cardiovascular disease risk factors.
- Mate: no benefit for reducing weight.

✖ *Likely to be ineffective or harmful*

- Guar gum: not effective for reducing body weight or feeling of hunger.
- Psyllium: no changes in body weight likely.
- Number ten: herbal combination preparation reported as not effective for reducing weight.

Conclusions

- Best evidence suggests that *Garcinica cambogia*, and hypnotherapy are likely to be beneficial but the evidence is not fully convincing
- Ephedra can reduce body weight but is associated with an increased risk of psychiatric, autonomic or gastrointestinal symptoms and heart palpitations. Allergic reactions should be considered. *Garcinia cambogia* and hypnotherapy are not associated with serious risks
- The risk–benefit balance is likely to be positive for *Garcinia cambogia* and hypnotherapy while there is a trade off between benefits and harms for ephedra
- Compared to conventional interventions, no CAM treatment is as beneficial as regular physical exercise and reduced energy intake

Further reading

Avenell A, Sattar N, Lean M. ABC of obesity. Management: Part I–behaviour change, diet, and activity. *BMJ* 2006; **333**:740–3.

Romero-Corral A, Montori VM, Somers VK *et al*. Association of bodyweight with total mortality and with cardiovascular events in coronary artery disease: a systematic review of cohort studies. *Lancet* 2006; **368**:666–78.

Neurology

Alzheimer's disease

Profile

Alzheimer's disease is a chronic, non-reversible, neurodegenerative disease characterized by an insidious onset and slow deterioration which involves impairments in speech, motor, personality, and executive functions. It is the most common type of dementia. Early symptoms such as deterioration of short-term memory become more pronounced as the condition advances and cognitive impairment extends to language, movements, recognition, decision-making, and planning. Neuronal atrophy occurs mainly in the temporoparietal and frontal cortices with deposition of amyloid plaques. The underlying cause is not known and there is currently no cure. It is primarily a clinical diagnosis and there are no tests to diagnose Alzheimer's disease conclusively.

Clinical bottom line

☺ *Beneficial:*

- Ginkgo (*Ginkgo biloba*): improvement of cognition and function.

☺ *Likely to be beneficial*

- Choto-san: Kampo medicine, may lead to global improvement.

☻ *Unknown effectiveness*

- Acupuncture: may improve symptoms yet few data available.
- Aromatherapy: may improve wellbeing yet few data available.
- *Huperzia serrata*: not enough data available.
- Lemon balm (*Melissa officinalis*): may improve cognitive function yet few data available.
- Massage: very limited amount of reliable evidence.
- Music therapy: may reduce agitation and aggressive behavior yet not enough data available.
- Omega-3 fatty acids: evidence to support its use is not strong enough.
- Sage (*Salvia officinalis*): may improve cognitive function yet few data available.
- Therapeutic touch: very limited amount of reliable evidence.
- Vitamin E: insufficient evidence of efficacy.

☠ *Likely to be ineffective or harmful*

- Electrostimulation: no effects on rest-activity rhythm and salivary cortisol.
- Ginseng (*Panax ginseng*): is likely to be ineffective for improving somatic symptoms, depression and anxiety.

Conclusions

- Best evidence suggests that *Ginkgo biloba* is beneficial for Alzheimer's disease. Choto-san is likely to be beneficial but the evidence is not fully convincing
- Adverse events and interactions need to be considered
- The risk–benefit balance for *Ginkgo biloba* is positive and likely to be positive for Choto-san
- *Ginkgo biloba* seems worth trying considering the limited options of conventional medicine

Further reading

Blennow K, de Leon MJ, Zetterberg H. Alzheimer's disease. *Lancet* 2006; **368**:387–403.

Ginkgo (*Ginkgo biloba*)

What is it?

A tree native to China, Korea and Japan. Leaves are used for medicinal purposes

How does it work?

Increase of microcirculatory blood flow, inhibition of platelet and erythrocyte aggregation, platelet-activating factor antagonism, free radical scavenging

How is it used?

Orally, as powdered extract

Are there any risks?

There is a possible risk of allergic reactions

Epilepsy

Profile

Epilepsy is characterized by seizures that can be classified as partial or generalized. A person is considered to have epilepsy if they have had 2 or more unprovoked seizures. Epilepsy is common, with an estimated prevalence in the developed world of 5–10 per 1000. About 3% of people will be given a diagnosis of epilepsy at some time in their lives. Epilepsy may be caused by various disorders of the brain and may include neonatal injuries, congenital or metabolic disorders, head injuries, tumours, or infections of the brain. The prognosis for most patients is good, about 70% go into remission, defined as being seizure-free for 5 years on or off treatment. CAM therapies often used include acupuncture, homeopathy, herbal medicine, osteopathy, chiropractic, biofeedback, relaxation, and yoga.

Clinical bottom line

😐 *Unknown effectiveness*

- Acupuncture: may reduce seizure frequency and duration, yet not enough data available.
- Biofeedback, EEG: not enough data available.
- Biofeedback, galvanic skin response: may reduce seizure frequency yet not enough data available.
- Cannabinoids: not enough data available.
- Meditation: data scarce and methodologically limited.
- Music therapy: may reduce seizure frequency yet not enough data available.
- Omega-3 fatty acids: may reduce seizure frequency and duration, yet not enough data available.
- Yoga: may reduce seizure frequency yet not enough data available.

😟 *Unlikely to be beneficial:*

- Relaxation: no effect on seizure frequency.

Conclusions

- No CAM is of proven effectiveness for epilepsy as a primary or adjunctive treatment
- The tested therapies and medicines seem relatively safe, but adverse events have been reported
- The risk–benefit balance fails to be positive for any CAM
- There are effective conventional options and CAM has little to offer for patients with epilepsy

Further reading

Pohlmann-Eden B, Beghi E, Camfield C, Camfield P. The first seizure and its management in adults and children. *BMJ* 2006; **332**:339–42.

Headache

Profile

Headache on at least 15 days per month for at least 6 months. Bilateral pain of a pressing tightening quality with mild or moderate intensity, possibly with nausea, photo-, or phonophobia. Other frequently used terms are tension headache, episodic tension-type headache, cephalgia, cephalea, and cerebralgia. About 1/3 of headache sufferers use CAM, mostly relaxation, chiropractic, herbal medicine, homeopathy, acupuncture.

Clinical bottom line

😀 Likely to be beneficial

- Biofeedback: results contradictory but recent rigorous trials suggest that it is an effective means of reducing pain.
- Hypnotherapy: results somewhat contradictory but majority of trials suggest benefit.
- Relaxation: results contradictory, the best studies tend to suggest a positive effect on pain.

😐 Unknown effectiveness

- Acupuncture: intensity and frequency, studies have generated contradictory results.
- Autogenic training: not superior to other interventions in terms of symptom control, data methodologically limited.
- Coshuguto: a Kampo (herbal) medicine, better than placebo in decreasing the number of episodes, but not enough data available.
- Guided imagery: might improve symptoms as an adjunct to standard care but more data needed.
- Massage therapy: not enough data available.
- Peppermint (*Mentha piperita*) oil (external): not enough data available.
- Reflexology: some encouraging data exist but are scarce and methodologically weak.
- Tai chi: might improve status and impact of tension headache but not enough data available.
- Therapeutic touch: preliminary data positive but analgesic effect short lived.
- Tiger balm (external): not enough data available.
- Trager approach: some reports are positive, but not enough data available.

☒ Likely to be ineffective or harmful

- Homeopathy: best studies fail to show beneficial effects.
- Spinal manipulation: results of effectiveness studies are contradictory, upper spinal manipulation has been associated with stroke and death.

Conclusions

- Biofeedback, hypnotherapy and relaxation are likely to be effective
- None of the treatments are associated with serious risks
- The risk–benefit balance could therefore turn out to be positive for these approaches
- Compared to conventional treatments the value of these CAM treatments is uncertain

Further reading

Bronfort G, Nilsson N, Haas M *et al.* Non-invasive physical treatments for chronic/recurrent headache. *Cochrane Database Syst Rev* 2004; **3**:CD001878.

Migraine

Profile

Primary headache disorder with recurring disabling pain, lasting 0.5–3 days sometimes with aura, nausea, photophobia and phonophobia. Other terms which are occasionally used include vascular, bilious, sick, or blind headache, haemicrania, haemiplegic, or ophthalmoplegic migraine. About 10–15% of the general population suffer from migraine. The aetiology is unknown and a genetic predisposition is being discussed. Often typical triggers exist which set off an episode. Many patients have tried CAM, particularly herbal medicine, spinal manipulation, acupuncture, homeopathy or reflexology. The domain of CAM is in prevention of migraine rather than in treating an acute attack.

Clinical bottom line

☺ Beneficial

- Biofeedback: reduces migraine frequency and improves self-efficacy.

☺ Likely to be beneficial

- Relaxation: seems to be useful for adults alone or in combination with biofeedback.

☻ Unknown effectiveness

- Acupuncture: may improve symptoms and number of migraine days but data often contradictory and methodologically weak.
- Butterbur (*Petasites hybridus*): preliminary data suggest reduction of attack frequency.
- Co-enzyme Q10: not enough data available.
- Feverfew: may reduce frequency or severity of pain but data are contradictory.
- Fish oil: not enough data available.
- Massage: preliminary data suggest reduction of frequency and improvement of sleep quality.
- Yoga: not enough data available.

☹ Unlikely to be beneficial

- Homeopathy: best evidence fails to show positive effects.

✖ Likely to be ineffective or harmful

- Spinal manipulation: not enough data available related to effectiveness, upper spinal manipulation has been associated with stroke and death.

Table 5.15 Systematic up-to-date review of treatment that is beneficial for migraine

Treatment	Source	No. of trials/ patients	Original conclusion
Biofeedback	*Pain* 2007; **128**: 111–27	N=55/n=2229	This meta-analysis documents medium effect sizes for the short- and long-term outcome of biofeedback for migraine in adults. Biofeedback significantly and substantially reduces the pain and psychological symptoms of highly chronified patients ...

Conclusions

- Biofeedback prevents migraine attacks. The evidence for relaxation is encouraging but more data are required to be sure
- When used correctly, biofeedback and relaxation are not associated with serious or frequent harm
- For biofeedback the risk–benefit balance seems positive: it is likely to be positive for relaxation
- Biofeedback has been shown to be similarly effective as propanolol

Further reading

Biondi DM. Physical treatments for headache: a structured review. *Headache* 2005; **45**:738–46.
Sandor PS, Afra J. Nonpharmacologic treatment of migraine. *Curr Pain Headache Rep* 2005; **9**:202–5.

Biofeedback

What is it?
A method using instruments to perceive body functions in order to control those functions

How does it work?
Modifications of physiological process at will

How is it used?
Used by a range of different types of practitioners in order to control autonomic functions and generate a relaxation response

Are there any risks?
Some reports suggest biofeedback can cause or aggravate psychological problems such as anxiety

Multiple sclerosis

Profile

Multiple sclerosis (synonym: encephalomyelitis disseminate) is a relatively common demyelinating disease affecting the central nervous system. Its aetiology is not known and is possibly multifactorial. An autoimmune disorder resulting from environmental stimuli in genetically susceptible individuals is being discussed. Early diagnosis can be difficult as symptoms vary greatly, are usually not specific and often fluctuate. Initially multiple sclerosis may mimic rheumatic conditions: later neurological deficits may dominate. Axonal loss leads to irreversible disability.

Clinical bottom line

😃 *Likely to be beneficial*

- Cannabis (*Cannabis sativa*): results are somewhat contradictory but some data suggest improvement in mobility, pain and sleep.

😐 *Unknown effectiveness*

- Acupuncture: paucity and poor quality of primary studies.
- Cannabis (*Cannabis sativa*): may reduce the number of incontinence episodes but not enough data available.
- Feldenkrais: preliminary results suggest stress and anxiety reduction but not enough data available.
- Fish oil: preliminary data suggest functional improvements.
- Ginkgo (*Ginkgo biloba*): preliminary data suggest it may improve fatigue, symptom severity and functionality but not cognitive function
- Imagery: not enough data available.
- Massage: preliminary results suggest improvements of anxiety and depression.
- Music therapy: strengthening of respiratory muscles through coordination of breath and speech, not enough data available.
- Neural therapy: preliminary data show a reduction of subjective symptoms.
- Reflexology: preliminary results suggest improvements of a range of symptoms such as motor sensory and urinary symptoms.
- Yoga: preliminary results suggest positive effects on fatigue.

😟 *Unlikely to be beneficial*

- Cannabis (*Cannabis sativa*): Unlikely to be beneficial in reducing tremor.

Conclusions

- No CAM has been shown to alter the natural course of multiple sclerosis. Cannabis may improve mobility, pain and sleep but more data are needed to be sure
- Cannabis is not free of risks but seem manageable with adequate supervision
- The risk–benefit balance for cannabis may turn out to be favourable, but more evidence is required

Further reading

Huntley A. A review of the evidence for efficacy of complementary and alternative medicines in MS. *Int MS J* 2006; **13**:4–12.

Parkinson's disease

Profile

Parkinson's disease is an incurable, neurodegenerative, progressive disease of unknown causes. Its symptoms include asymmetrical bradykinesia, hypokinesia, rigidity, and tremor. There is a progressive loss of dopamine-producing cells in the brain-stem. The overall age-adjusted prevalence is around 1.5%, rising in older age groups. The treatment is largely symptomatic and aims at compensating for the lack of dopamine. Many Parkinson patients try CAM, mostly for symptom control.

Clinical bottom line

😔 *Unknown effectiveness*

- Acupuncture: data contradictory and scarce.
- Alexander technique: preliminary data suggest reduction of disability.
- Antioxidants: data contradictory.
- Co-enzyme Q10: some studies suggest high doses (1200mg daily) slow progressive deterioration of function but not enough data available.
- Music therapy: preliminary data suggest positive effects on motor, affective, and behavioural functions.
- *Mucuna pruriens* is a herbal medicine from the Ayurvedic tradition which is a natural source of L-dopa: preliminary data encouraging.
- Qigong: preliminary data suggest improvement of motor symptoms.

😞 *Unlikely to be beneficial*

- Cannabis (*Cannabis sativa*): unlikely to reduce tremor.

Conclusions

- No CAM is of proven effectiveness for Parkinson's disease
- The risks of the tested treatments are small
- A risk–benefit analysis fails to be positive
- Compared to conventional therapy, CAM has little to offer for Parkinson patients

Further reading

Chung V, Liu L, Bian Z, Zhao Z et al. Efficacy and safety of herbal medicines for idiopathic Parkinson's disease: a systematic review. *Mov Disord* 2006; **21**:1709–15.

Horstink M, Tolosa E, Bonuccelli U et al. Review of the therapeutic management of Parkinson's disease. Report of a joint task force of the European Federation of Neurological Societies (EFNS) and the Movement Disorder Society-European Section (MDS-ES). Part II: late (complicated) Parkinson's disease. *Eur J Neurol* 2006; **13**:1186–1202.

Oncology

Cancer

Profile

A diverse group of neoplastic disorders characterized by uncontrolled cell growth at various sites in the body. Cancer is one of the leading causes of death worldwide. It also is a frequent reason for patients to turn to CAM—virtually all cancer patients consider trying CAM and most use it.

Prevention

Clinical bottom line

😊 *Beneficial*

- *Allium* vegetables (e.g. garlic): regular intake reduces risk, particularly of gastrointestinal cancers.
- Exercise: reduces risk of colon and breast cancer.
- Green tea (*Camellia sinensis*): regular intake reduces risk of cancer of the upper digestive tract and of the breast.
- Tomato (lycopene): regular intake of tomato-based products reduces risk of prostate cancer.

😊 *Likely to be beneficial*

- Phytoestrogens: preliminary data suggest risk reduction for some forms of malignancies, particularly prostate cancer.

😐 *Unknown effectiveness*

- Antioxidants: data contradictory.
- Calcium: effect on colorectal cancer risk is small.
- Dietary fibre: data inconclusive.
- Fish oil: not enough data available.
- Ginseng (*Panax ginseng*): not enough data available.
- Vegetarianism: data contradictory.

Conclusions

- Regular exercise and regular intake of allium vegetables, green tea and tomato products and possibly phytoestrogens reduces risk of certain cancers
- None of these interventions carry high risks
- Their risk–benefit balance is therefore positive
- These interventions may supplement conventional risk reduction strategies

Treatment

Clinical bottom line

😐 *Unknown effectiveness*

- Asian mixtures: numerous mixtures exist but independent replications are rare.
- Beta glucan: not enough data available.

- Essiac: no controlled clinical studies.
- Gerson diet: no reliable data available.
- Hydrazine sulphate: not enough data available.
- Macrobiotic diet: no reliable studies.
- Melatonin: not enough data available.
- Mistletoe (*Viscum album*): clinical studies contradictory.
- Reishi (*Ganoderma lucidum*): not enough data available.
- Ukrain: the trial data are encouraging for a range of cancers but the studies are methodologically weak.

✖ *Likely to be ineffective or harmful*
- Di Bella therapy: some studies suggest worse survival rates.
- Laetrile: no evidence of effectiveness and potential for serious harm.
- Shark cartilage: best clinical studies fail to show an effect on survival.
- Support group therapy: best studies fail to show an effect on survival.
- Thymus gland extract: no good evidence for effectiveness.

Conclusions

- No CAM therapy has been shown to change the natural history of any cancer
- Some treatments carry considerable risks
- The risk–benefit balance fails to be positive
- Compared to conventional treatments CAM has nothing to offer for treating cancer

Palliation

Clinical bottom line

☺ *Beneficial*
- Aromatherapy: improves wellbeing and reduces anxiety.
- Exercise: regular exercise reduces severity of adverse effects caused by conventional treatments.
- Massage: improves wellbeing.

☺ *Likely to be beneficial*
- Acupuncture: some trial show an effect on nausea but other studies contradict these findings (📖 see also chemotherapy-related nausea and vomiting p.300).
- Enzymes: may reduce adverse effects of conventional therapies.
- Factor AF2, an extract from the spleen and liver of sheep embryos and lamb: may reduce myelotixicity of conventional treatments.
- Hypnotherapy: relief of chemotherapy-induced nausea and vomiting.
- Music therapy for psychological problems: preliminary data positive.
- Relaxation for pain or improvement of anxiety and increase in wellbeing: most studies demonstrate positive effects.

☹ *Unknown effectiveness*
- Acupuncture: trial results for pain and xerostomia contradictory.
- Asian herbal mixtures: preliminary results are encouraging scarce.
- Cannabinoids: results on pain-control, appetite, or quality of life are inconsistent.

- Co-enzyme Q10: may reduce toxicity of some conventional treatments but data scarce and methodologically limited.
- Fish oil: data contradictory for prevention of cachexia.
- Ginkgo (*Ginkgo biloba*): for lymphoedema, not enough data available.
- Ginseng (*Panax ginseng*) for fatigue and quality of life but not enough data available.
- Homeopathy: some encouraging but methodologically limited data for a range of problems.
- Hypnotherapy: more data required for the relief of pain and fatigue.
- Marigold (*Calendula officinalis*) for radiation-induced dermatitis in breast cancer: not enough data available.
- Spiritual healing: for reduction of anxiety and increase in wellbeing but studies methodologically weak.

🙁 *Unlikely to be beneficial*
- Reflexology: results mixed but best study was negative for improving quality of life.

☒ *Likely to be ineffective or harmful*
- Aloe vera: no effects on radiation-induced skin irritation and oral mucositis.
- Black cohosh (*Actaea racemosa*): results regarding hot flushes contradictory and has been associated with liver damage.
- Cranberry (*Vaccinium macrocarpon*): no efficacy for prostate cancer symptoms.
- Phytoestrogens: no efficacy for hot flushes.
- Soy products: no efficacy for hot flushes.

Table 5.16 Systematic up-to-date review of treatment that is beneficial for cancer palliation

Treatment	Source	No. of trials/ patients	Original conclusion
Aromatherapy	*Cochrane Database Syst Rev* 2004; **3**:CD002287	N=8/n=357	Short-term benefits on psychological wellbeing

Conclusions

- Aromatherapy, exercise, and massage are effective means of palliation and a range of other treatments are likely to be beneficial
- Their risks are minimal
- The risk–benefit balance is positive for aromatherapy, exercise, and massage and likely to be positive for a number of other treatments
- These treatments are useful adjuncts in cancer palliation

Further reading

Gerber B, Scholz C, Reimer T, Briese V, Janni W. Complementary and alternative therapeutic approaches in patients with early breast cancer: a systematic review. *Breast Cancer Res Treat* 2006; **95**:199–209.

Hercberg S, Czernichow S, Galan P. Antioxidant vitamins and minerals in prevention of cancers: lessons from the SU.VI.MAX study. *Br J Nutr* 2006; **96**(1):S28–30.

Mansky PJ, Wallerstedt DB. Complementary medicine in palliative care and cancer symptom management. *Cancer J* 2006; **12**: 425–31.

Vickers AJ, Kuo J, Cassileth BR. Unconventional anticancer agents: a systematic review of clinical trials. *J Clin Oncol* 2006; **24**:136–140.

Aromatherapy

What is it?
Medicinal use of essential oils

How does it work?
In theory, scents could alter brain function or oils could act through pharmacological properties of absorbed substances

How is it used?
Usually through gentle massage (which could have relaxing effects in itself)

Are there any risks?
Negligible in most cases

Exercise

What is it?
Physical exercise is the performance of activity to develop or maintain physical fitness and overall health. Frequent and regular physical exercise is an important component in the prevention of diseases such as heart disease, cardiovascular disease, type 2 diabetes, and obesity

How does it work?
Healthy weight balance; building and maintaining healthy bone density, muscle strength, and joint mobility; promoting physiological and psychological well-being; strengthening the immune system; improving cognitive function

How is it used?
It is best to exercise regularly 30 minutes, 5 times weekly (e.g. brisk walk)

Are there any risks?
Delayed muscle soreness, sprains and falls may occur. A doctor should be consulted before taking up an exercise program or radical changes are made to an existing exercise regimen

Garlic (Allium sativum)

What is it?
Common culinary plant (bulb)

How does it work?
Most likely through a range of effects that act synergistically

How is it used?
As food stuff or dietary supplement for a range of therapeutic preventative indications

Are there any risks?
Some risks are known but manageable

Massage

What is it?
A method of manipulating the soft tissue of whole body areas using pressure and traction

How does it work?
The circulation of blood and lymph is generally enhanced, resulting in increased oxygen supply and allegedly in the removal of waste products

How is it used?
The duration of individual treatment sessions varies, but will typically be about 30 minutes. Usually, 1–2 sessions weekly for a treatment period of 4–8 weeks

Are there any risks?
Few risks involved

Tomato (Lycopersicon esculentum)

What is it?
Tomato is a plant in the Solanaceae or nightshade family. The fruits are used

How does it work?
Lycopene, a caroteniod found in tomatoes, is thought to have cancer preventing effects

How is it used?
Consumption of tomato based products. Cooking releases lycopene.

Are there any risks?
No serious adverse events known

Otorhinolaryngology

Allergic rhinitis (seasonal)

Profile

Seasonal allergic rhinitis, also called pollinosis, hay fever, or nasal allergy is a complex of symptoms that may affect several organ systems. It occurs after exposure to the pollens of specific seasonal plants in people who are allergic to these substances. Symptoms will consist of seasonal sneezing, nasal itching, nasal blockage, and watery nasal discharge. Eye symptoms (red eyes, itchy eyes, and tearing) are common. Prevalence of CAM use in patients with allergies is high and hay fever is the allergy most commonly treated with CAM.

Clinical bottom line

☺ *Likely to be beneficial*

- Butterbur (*Petasites hybridus*): superior to placebo and equal to non-sedative antihistamines.

☹ *Unknown effectiveness*

- Acupuncture: conflicting data for both prevention and treatment.
- Chinese herbal medicine: different formulae tested, not enough data available.
- Homeopathy: data conflicting for preparations of *Galphimia glauca*, not enough data available for *Luffa compositum* Heel and other homeopathic remedies.
- Hypnosis: improvements reported with self-hypnosis but not enough data available.
- Nettle (*Urtica dioica*): higher global ratings of symptom improvement but only few data with methodological limitations.
- *Tinaspora cordifolia*: might decrease symptoms but not enough data available.
- Vitamin E: might reduce nasal symptom scores when administered in addition to regular antiallergic treatment, only few data available.

✗ *Likely to be ineffective or harmful*

- Grape seed (*Vitis vinifera*): no evidence of efficacy reported.
- Royal jelly: no effect on occurrence or severity of symptoms.

Table 5.17 Systematic up-to-date review of treatments that are likely to be beneficial for seasonal allergic rhinitis

Treatment	Source	No. of trials/ patients	Original conclusion
Butterbur (*Petasites hybridus*)	*Ann Allergy, Asthma Immunology* 2008 (in press)	N=6/n=720	There is encouraging evidence suggesting that *P. hybridus* may be an effective herbal treatment for seasonal (intermittent) allergic rhinitis

Conclusions

- Butterbur is likely to be effective
- It is not associated with any serious risks but allergic reactions to butterbur are possible
- The risk–benefit balance for butterbur is likely to be positive
- Butterbur might be equally effective as fexofenadine and cetirizine

Further reading

Passalacqua G, Bousquet PJ, Carlsen KH et al. ARIA update: I–Systematic review of complementary and alternative medicine for rhinitis and asthma. J Allergy Clin Immunol 2006; **117**:1054–62.

Loss of hearing

Profile

Loss of hearing is a full or partial decrease in the ability to detect sounds. The two main categories are: 1) conductive hearing loss, which is due to mechanical problems in the outer or middle ear at the level of the ossicles or eardrum and 2) sensorineural hearing loss, which is due to dysfunction in the cochlea, most often at the level of the sound receptor—the hair cell. Causes include long-term exposure to environmental noise, mumps, measles, and meningitis. Prevention of hearing loss is the main objective in its management. Herbal medicines are often used for this condition.

Clinical bottom line

☺ *Likely to be beneficial*
- Ginkgo (*Ginkgo biloba*): may improve hearing threshold.
- Folic acid: may slow age-related hearing loss.

☹ *Unknown effectiveness*
- Acupuncture: data scarce and contradictory.
- Homeopathy: not enough data available.
- Puerarin: not enough data available for this constituent of kudzu (*Pueraria lobata*).
- Chinese herbal mixtures: not enough data available.

Conclusions

- No CAM is of proven effectiveness for hearing loss. Ginkgo and folic acid are likely to be beneficial but the evidence is not fully convincing
- No serious risks have been reported but adverse events, allergic reactions and drug interactions should be considered
- The risk–benefit balance might be positive for Ginkgo and folic acid
- There are effective conventional options for patients with loss of hearing

Further reading

Gates GA, Mills JH. Presbycusis. *Lancet* 2005; **366**:1111–20.
Smith RJ, Bale JF Jr, White KR. Sensorineural hearing loss in children. *Lancet* 2005; **365**:879–90.

Otitis media

Profile

Infection, usually bacterial by nature, of the middle ear is common, particularly in children. The main symptom is piercing, local pain. Fever occurs frequently. Close to 100% of children will have experienced otitis media by the time they reach 7 years of age. The condition can become recurrent or chronic. Conventional therapy is often claimed to be unnecessary if CAM is employed. Popular CAM options include homeopathic and herbal medicines.

Clinical bottom line

😑 *Unknown effectiveness*

- Anthroposophical medicine: data methodologically too weak to be reliable.
- Chinese herbal mixtures: various mixtures have been tested but trials methodologically weak and scarce.
- Herbal ear drops: several mixtures have been tested (e.g. Otikon, Otic solution) with encouraging results but more data required.
- Xylitol, a birch derived polyol sugar for oral consumption: seems to have antibacterial effects, preliminary data encouraging.

🗯 *Likely to be ineffective or harmful*

- Homeopathy: the most reliable trials fail to demonstrate effectiveness.
- Spinal manipulation: the trial data collectively fail to show effectiveness, upper spinal manipulation has been associated with stroke and death.

Conclusions

- No CAM have been proven to be effective
- The treatments in question seem relatively safe
- The risk–benefit balance fails to be positive for any CAM
- Compared with conventional treatments (e.g. pain control and, if necessary, antibiotics) CAM has little to offer for sufferers from otitis media

Further reading

Rovers MM, Schilder AG, Zielhuis GA, Rosenfeld RM. Otitis media. *Lancet* 2004; **363**:465–73.

Tinnitus

Profile

Hearing a sound in the absence of external noise can be distressing. As tinnitus often proves to be resistant to conventional treatments many sufferers turn to CAM. Popular approaches include acupuncture, *Ginkgo biloba*, and hypnotherapy.

Clinical bottom line

☺ *Likely to be beneficial*

- Hypnotherapy: seems to reduce the loudness of the experienced sounds.

☻ *Unknown effectiveness*

- Acupuncture: the most rigorous studies were negative but more recently trial results have been more encouraging.
- Biofeedback: data scant, contradictory, and methodologically flawed
- Chinese herbal formulae: many formulae exist and for none is the evidence convincing.

☹ *Unlikely to be beneficial*

- Ginkgo (*Ginkgo biloba*): Unlikely to be beneficial.

☒ *Likely to be ineffective or harmful*

- Cognitive behavioural therapy: seems not effective for reducing loudness of experienced sounds.
- Homeopathy: scant data failed to show any effect beyond placebo.
- Melatonin: not better than placebo.
- Yoga: trials do not show any beneficial effects.
- Zinc: not better than placebo.

Conclusions

- Hypnotherapy may be effective in reducing the loudness of the experienced sound but more trials of a higher quality are needed to be sure
- Few risks are associated with hypnotherapy
- The risk–benefit ratio is likely to be positive for hypnotherapy
- Neither conventional nor CAM approaches seems to control tinnitus convincingly and reliably

Further reading

Waddell A. Tinnitus. *Clin Evid* 2005; **14**:703–11.

Psychiatry

Anxiety

Profile

A complex combination of emotions such as fear, apprehension, and worry. Physical symptoms include amongst others, palpitations, nausea and chest pain. The International Classification of Disease differentiates phobic anxiety disorders, other anxiety disorders, obsessive-compulsive disorders, adjustment disorders, dissociative disorders, and other neurotic disorders. About half of all sufferers try CAM, particularly relaxation, herbal medicines, music therapy, hypnotherapy, meditation, and yoga.

Clinical bottom line

☺ Beneficial

- Massage: decreases anxiety in a variety of settings.
- Music therapy: reduces anxiety in hospitalized patients.
- Relaxation: certain relaxation techniques reduce trait anxiety.

☺ Likely to be beneficial

- Acupuncture: preliminary data suggest a relaxation response after acupuncture.
- Aromatherapy: effects are short-term and thus of questionable clinical relevance.
- Guided imagery: encouraging evidence e.g. in cancer patients.
- Hypnotherapy: encouraging data, particularly for phobias.
- Meditation: encouraging evidence for trait anxiety.

⊕ Trade off between benefits and harms

- Kava (*Piper methysticum*): anxiolytic effects are well documented but suspicion of hepatotoxicity.

☺ Unknown effectiveness

- Autogenic training: preliminary data are encouraging but most studies methodologically weak.
- Biofeedback: results contradictory.
- Breathing exercises: dental anxiety, not enough data available.
- Chamomile (*Matricaria recutita*): not enough data available.
- Exercise: not enough data available.
- Ginkgo (*Ginkgo biloba*): preliminary data suggest positive effects in generalized anxiety disorder
- Lemon balm (*Melissa officinalis*): not enough data available.
- Passion flower (*Passiflora incarnata*): not enough data available.
- Reflexology: anxiety in cancer patients, not enough data available.
- Reiki: studies are methodologically weak not enough data available.
- Tai chi: anxiolytyic activity of regular tai chi but not enough data available.
- Therapeutic touch: encouraging but methodologically weak data.
- Yoga: studies tend to generate positive findings particularly with obsessive compulsive disorders, but most are methodologically weak.

😞 *Unlikely to be beneficial*
- Homeopathy: majority of trials were negative.

☒ *Likely to be ineffective or harmful*
- Chiropractic: no effect on state anxiety.
- Flower remedies: best studies fail to show effect.
- Valerian (*Valeriana officinalis*): efficacy not demonstrated.

Table 5.19 Systematic up-to-date reviews of treatments that are beneficial or likely to be beneficial for anxiety

Treatment	Source	No. of trials/ patients	Original conclusion
Aromatherapy	*Br J Gen Pract* 2000; **50**:493–6	N=12/n=1463	Aromatherapy massage has a mild, transient anxiolytic effect
Guided imagery	*Psychooncology* 2005; **14**:607–17	N=6/n=not available	Three studies reported significant differences in measures of anxiety, comfort or emotional response to chemo-therapy
Meditation	*J Altern Complement Med* 2006; **12**: 817–32	N=20/n=958	Benefit was demon-strated for mood and anxiety disorders
Music therapy	*J Adv Nurs* 2002; **37**:8–18	N=12/n=not available	This systematic review of music for adults during hospitalization clearly demonstrates its effectiveness for the reduction of anxiety during normal care delivery

Conclusions

- Massage, music therapy, relaxation, and kava are demonstrably effective in reducing anxiety; a range of other CAM therapies are likely to be effective
- Kava has been associated with liver damage, none of the other treatments are associated with serious risks
- The risk–benefit balance for massage, music therapy, and relaxation is positive and likely to be positive for acupuncture, aromatherapy, guided imagery, hypnotherapy, and meditation
- There are, of course, highly effective treatments in conventional medicine. Most are, however, burdened with significant safety issues. The relative value of CAM requires equivalence studies, which currently are not available

Further reading

Ernst E. Herbal remedies for anxiety–a systematic review of controlled clinical trials. *Phytomedicine* 2006; **13**:205–8.

Jorm AF, Christensen H, Griffiths KM *et al.* Effectiveness of complementary and self-help treatments for anxiety disorders. *Med J Aust* 2004; **181**(7):S29–46.

Massage

What is it?
A method of manipulating the soft tissue of whole body areas using pressure and traction

How does it work?
The circulation of blood and lymph is generally enhanced, resulting in increased oxygen supply and allegedly in the removal of waste products

How is it used?
The duration of individual treatment sessions varies, but will typically be about 30 minutes. Usually, 1–2 sessions weekly for a treatment period of 4–8 weeks

Are there any risks?
Few risks involved

Music therapy

What is it?
The use of music for therapeutic purposes

How does it work?
Sensations that accompany music therapy may activate limbic or other areas of the brain related to the reward and motivation circuitry (limbic-cortical circuits)

How is it used?
Depending on the condition, either receptive (listening to music played by the therapist or recorded music) or active music therapy (patients are involved in the music-making) is used

Are there any risks?
No risks have been reported

Relaxation therapy

What is it?
Techniques for eliciting the 'relaxation response' of the autonomic nervous system

How does it work?
Progressive muscle relaxation elicits the relaxation response, resulting in the normalizing of blood supply to the muscles, decreases in oxygen consumption, heart rate, respiration and skeletal muscle activity and increases in skin resistance and alpha brain waves. Other relaxation techniques involve passive muscle relaxation, refocusing or breathing

How is it used?
Several months of daily practice is needed in order to be able to evoke the relaxation response

Are there any risks?
None known

Attention deficit hyperactivity disorder

Profile

Attention deficit hyperactivity disorder (ADHD) is a persistent pattern of inattention and hyperactivity and impulsivity that is more frequent and severe than is typically observed in people at a comparable level of development. Symptoms of ADHD must be present for at least 6 months, observed before the age of 7 years, and clinically important impairment in social, academic, or occupational functioning must exist. DSM-IV prevalence estimates among US school children are 3–5%: other estimates vary from 1.7–16.0%. More than 70% of hyperactive children may continue to meet criteria for ADHD in adolescence, and up to 65% of adolescents may continue to meet such criteria in adulthood. The underlying causes of ADHD are not known. CAM treatments include dietary supplements and homeopathy.

Clinical bottom line

☹ *Unknown effectiveness*

- EEG biofeedback: may lead to clinical improvement yet not enough data available.
- French maritime bark (*Pinus pinaster*): may improve symptoms but data contradictory.
- Homeopathy: data scarce and contradictory.
- Jiangqian: not enough data available for this Chinese herbal remedy.
- Massage: not enough data available.
- Music therapy: not enough data available.
- Neurofeedback: not enough data available.
- Omega-3 fatty acids: data scarce and contradictory.
- Stress management: no effect on self-concept, control and coping skills yet not enough data available.
- Yoga: may improve symptoms but data scarce.

☹ *Unlikely to be beneficial*

- Bach flower remedies.

Conclusions

- No CAM is of proven effectiveness for ADHD
- For omega-3 fatty acids vitamin D hypervitaminosis has been reported. Allergic reactions and herb–drug interactions are potentially serious risks. Other treatments seem relatively safe
- The risk–benefit balance fails to be positive for any CAM
- There are conventional options which are likely beneficial and CAM seems to have little to offer for patients with ADHD

Further reading

Biederman J, Faraone SV. Attention-deficit hyperactivity disorder. *Lancet* 2005; **366**:237–48.

Depression

Profile

Mild-to-moderate depression is defined as persistent low mood, loss of interest and reduced energy leading to functional impairment. In severe depression there is also agitation or psychosomatic retardation and marked somatic symptoms. Depression is one of the most common affective disorders and is associated with a high burden of suffering. It also is an important risk factor for suicide. Depression is among the most common reasons for trying CAM. The most widely used treatments include herbal medicine and relaxation.

Clinical bottom line

:☻: *Beneficial*

- St John's wort (*Hypericum perforatum*): effective for mild-to-moderate depression.

☻ *Likely to be beneficial*

- Autogenic training: trial data are encouraging but more rigorous studies are required.
- Massage: studies are positive but not fully convincing.
- Relaxation: trial data suggests that it is similarly effective as cognitive behaviour therapy.
- Yoga: several trials have shown reduction of depressive symptoms.

☻ *Trade off between benefits and harms*

- Black cohosh (*Actaea racemosa*): seems to improve depression in menopausal women but has been associated with liver damage.

☻ *Unknown effectiveness*

- Acupressure: may improve symptoms of depression yet not enough data available.
- Acupuncture: evidence inconclusive.
- Aromatherapy: not enough data available.
- *Echium amoenum*: not enough data available.
- Fish oil: the evidence is limited and heterogeneous.
- Guided imagery: preliminary evidence is encouraging but not enough data available.
- Hypnotherapy: may improve symptoms of depression but not enough data available.
- Lavender (*Lavendula angustifolia*): not enough data available.
- Magnetic stimulation: not enough data available.
- Mindfulness-based stress reduction: may improve depression yet not enough data available.
- Music therapy: some encouraging results regarding psychological parameters but not enough data available.
- Reiki: not enough data available.
- Saffron (*Crocus saticus*): not enough data available.
- Zinc: not enough data available.

⚔ *Likely to be ineffective or harmful*
● Ginkgo (*Ginkgo biloba*): trial data fail to suggest effectiveness.

Table 5.20 Systematic up-to-date reviews of treatments that are beneficial or likely to be beneficial for depression

Treatment	Source	No. of trials/ patients	Original conclusion
Autogenic training	*Appl Psychophysiol Biofeedback* 2002; **27**:45–98	N=3/n=105	Positive effects (medium range) of AT and of AT versus control in the meta-analysis of at least 3 studies were found for […] mild-to-moderate depression/dysthymia
St John's wort	*Cochrane Database Syst Rev* 2005; **2**:CD000448	N=37/n=4925	Overall, hypericum extracts improved symptoms more than placebo, and similarly to synthetic antidepressants in adults with mild to moderate depression. However, pooled analysis of six recent, large, more precise trials that included only patients suffering from major depression showed only minimal benefits compared with placebo

Conclusions

● St John's wort is effective for mild-to-moderate depression. Autogenic training, black cohosh, massage, relaxation, and yoga are likely to be effective
● A significant risk of herb–drug interactions with St John's wort exists, black cohosh has been associated with liver damage, the other above therapies are not associated with serious risks
● The risk–benefit balance for St John's wort is positive if interactions are avoided and likely to be positive for the other above treatments
● St John's wort seems to be as effective as conventional antidepressants for mild-to-moderate depression

Further reading

Werneke U, Turner T, Priebe S. Complementary medicines in psychiatry: review of effectiveness and safety. *Br J Psychiatry* 2006; **188**:109–21.

St John's wort (*Hypericum perforatum*)

What is it?
Common plant with long history of medicinal use

How does it work?
As conventional antidepressants, e.g. selective serotonin reuptake inhibitors

How is it used?
Oral food supplement

Are there any risks?
Interactions with many prescription drugs

Drug/alcohol dependence

Profile

Drug or alcohol dependence (addiction, chemical dependence, substance abuse, substance use disorder) is the continued or increasing use of a chemical substance, to the extent of having negative consequences upon a person's life, in order to avoid physical or psychological withdrawal symptoms. The most frequently used CAM therapies are acupuncture and hypnotherapy.

Clinical bottom line

☺ *Likely to be beneficial*
- Biofeedback: alcohol dependence, control over drinking.

😐 *Unknown effectiveness*
- Acupressure: substance abuse, not enough data available.
- Acupuncture: data conflicting for alcohol and heroin dependence.
- Banxia Houpu: Chinese herbal decoction for heroin dependence, not enough data available.
- Chinese herbs: used rectally, data scarce and methodologically weak.
- Kudzu (*Pueria lobata*): Chinese herbal remedy, data conflicting.
- Passionflower (*Passiflora incarnata*): opiate dependence, not enough data available.
- Qigong: reduced withdrawal symptoms during detoxification of heroin addicts but not enough data available.
- Relaxation: might improve sleep pattern but too few data available
- Therapeutic touch: pregnant women with chemical dependency, too few data available.
- WeiniCom: Chinese herbal compound, not enough data available.
- Yoga: methadone maintenance therapy, too few data available.

😟 *Unlikely to be beneficial*
- Cranial electrostimulation: cocaine/opiate dependence.
- *Ginkgo biloba*: unlikely to be beneficial in cocaine dependence.
- Hypnotherapy: alcohol-dependence.

☒ *Likely to be ineffective or harmful*
- Acupuncture: no evidence that it is effective for cocaine dependence.
- Relaxation: not effective for drug withdrawal.

Conclusions

- Biofeedback is likely to be effective in alcohol dependence
- No serious risks have been reported for it
- The risk–benefit balance for biofeedback seems positive
- Inconsistent findings exist for comparison of biofeedback with other treatments or standard care

Further reading

Dean AJ. Natural and complementary therapies for substance use disorders. *Curr Opin Psychiatry* 2005; **18**:271–6.

Prendergast M, Podus D, Finney J *et al.* Contingency management for treatment of substance use disorders: a meta-analysis. *Addiction* 2006; **101**:1546–60.

Work Group on Substance Abuse Disorders, *et al.* Treatment of patients with substance use disorder, second edn. American Psychiatric Association. *Am J Psychiatry* 2006; **163**(8 Suppl):5–82.

Schizophrenia

Profile

Schizophrenia is a chronic and disabling brain disorder. It is characterized by auditory hallucinations, delusions, thought disorder, demotivation, self neglect, and reduced emotion, and by the cognitive symptoms of problems with attention, memory, and executive functions that allow people to plan and organize. People are defined as being resistant to standard antipsychotic drugs if, over the preceding 5 years, they have not had a clinically important improvement in symptoms after 2–3 regimens of treatment with standard antipsychotic drugs for at least 6 weeks and they have had no period of good functioning. Supplements as well as mind–body therapies have been tried.

Clinical bottom line

😊 *Likely to be beneficial*

- Music therapy: may improve global state when administered in addition to standard care.

😐 *Unknown effectiveness*

- Acupuncture: data are inconclusive.
- Art therapy: might improve adherence to therapy but not enough data available.
- Chinese herbal medicine: may be beneficial when combined with antipsychotics but not enough data available.
- Ginkgo (*Ginkgo biloba*): administered as an adjunct to may enhance efficiency of antipsychotics but not enough studies available.
- Hypnosis: data scarce and methodologically weak.
- Polyunsaturated fatty acids: data are inconclusive.

Table 5.21 Systematic up-to-date review of treatment that is likely to be beneficial for schizophrenia

Treatment	Source	No. of trials/ patients	Original conclusion
Music therapy	*Cochrane Database Syst Rev* 2005; **2**: CD004025	N=4/n=266	Music therapy as an addition to standard care helps people with schizophrenia to improve their global state and may also improve mental state and functioning

Conclusions

- There is encouraging evidence for music therapy in addition to antipsychotics
- Music therapy is virtually risk-free
- The risk–benefit balance for music therapy as an adjunct is likely to be positive
- There is no curative CAM treatment of schizophrenia and it should only used in addition to antipsychotic treatment

Further reading

Werneke U, Turner T, Priebe S. Complementary medicines in psychiatry: review of effectiveness and safety. *Br J Psychiatry* 2006; **188**:109–21.

Respiratory diseases

Asthma

Profile

Asthma is a common condition caused by airflow obstruction due to constriction of the airways and hyper-responsiveness of the bronchi. Most asthma sufferers are atopic. Symptoms include dyspnœa, wheezing, chronic cough, and tightness of the chest. Chronic asthma can be defined as asthma requiring maintenance treatments. There are marked regional differences but, overall, the prevalence of asthma is about 10%. Up to 70% of all asthma patients have been reported to use CAM. Popular treatments are special breathing techniques, relaxation, homeopathy and herbal medicines.

Clinical bottom line

😊 *Likely to be beneficial*

- Biofeedback: results uniformly show improvement of symptoms or less need for medication. Unfortunately only few studies exist.
- Breathing exercises: several breathing techniques have been developed, e.g. physiotherapy; results are encouraging and suggest better control of dyspnœa.
- Buteyko breathing: even though results are not entirely uniform they are on balance encouraging.

😐 *Unknown effectiveness*

- Acupuncture: results are inconsistent.
- AKL1: a herbal mixture fails to show effectiveness yet few trials available.
- Amrita bindu, Ayurvedic herbal mixture: not enough data available.
- Autogenic training: results conflicting.
- Butterbur (*Petasites hybridus*): not enough data available.
- Cannabis (*Cannabis sativa*): not enough data available.
- Chinese herbal medicine: most studies methodologically weak.
- Ding Chuan Tang, a Chinese herbal mixture: not enough data available.
- Fish oil: data inconsistent.
- Hypnotherapy: results are encouraging but scarce.
- Indian frankincense (*Boswellia serrata*): not enough data available.
- Ivy (*Hedera helix*): not enough data available.
- Magnesium: not enough data available.
- Massage: not enough data available.
- Meditation: not enough data available.
- *Picrorrizia kurroa*: not enough data available.
- Propolis: not enough data available.
- Relaxation: trial data methodologically weak.
- Saibuko-to: not enough data available.
- Vitamin C: evidence is insufficient.
- Yoga: results contradictory.

😞 *Unlikely to be beneficial*
- Chiropractic: most trials fail to indicate effectiveness.
- Homeopathy: the best evidence shows no effectiveness for lung function and attack frequency.
- Reflexology: best studies fail to indicate effectiveness for attack frequency.
- Selenium: best evidence does not indicate effectiveness.
- Spiritual healing: the best evidence shows no effectiveness.

Table 5.22 Systematic up-to-date review of treatment that is likely to be beneficial for asthma

Treatment	Source	No. of trials/ patients	Original conclusion
Breathing techniques	*Eur Resp J* 2000; **15**:969–972	N=5/n=150	Breathing exercises appear to be promising

Conclusions

- Biofeedback and breathing techniques (including Buteyko) are likely to be beneficial
- The risks of these treatments are minor
- The risk–benefit balance is likely to be positive for these therapies
- CAM therapies should not be used as alternatives to conventional treatments which are clearly more effective

Further reading

Passalacqua G, Bousquet PJ, Carlsen KH et al. ARIA update: I–Systematic review of complementary and alternative medicine for rhinitis and asthma. *J Allergy Clin Immunol* 2006; **117**:1054–62.

Yorke J, Fleming SL, Shuldham C. Psychological interventions for adults with asthma: A systematic review. *Respir Med* 2007; **101**:1–14.

Cystic fibrosis

Profile

One in 22 Europeans carry one gene responsible for this common, incurable, fatal, and inherited (autosomal recessive) disease. Progressive disability is caused mostly by recurrent lung infections resulting in chronic dyspnoea. Most patients die from lung failure between the age of 20–30 years. Even though pulmonary problems are the most prominent, cystic fibrosis affects the whole body. Popular CAM approaches include massage and herbal medicine.

Clinical bottom line

😐 *Unknown effectiveness*

- Acupuncture: preliminary data suggest positive effects on pain but not enough data available.
- Antioxidants: beta-carotene or selenium reduce oxidative stress which might preserve lung function but data not uniform and scarce.
- Fish oil: some studies suggest positive effects on lung function and need for antibiotics but more data needed.
- Massage therapy: may assist conventional treatments (e.g. in terms of reducing anxiety) but data scarce.
- Music therapy: seems promising as an adjunct to conventional therapies.

Conclusions

- No CAM is of proven effectiveness in cystic fibrosis as a primary or adjunctive treatment
- The tested treatments seem relatively safe
- The risk–benefit balance fails to be positive for any CAM
- Compared to a multidisciplinary conventional approach, CAM has little to offer for cystic fibrosis patients

Further reading

Ratjen F, Doring G. Cystic fibrosis. *Lancet* 2003; **361**:681–9.

Chronic obstructive pulmonary disease

Profile

Chronic obstructive pulmonary disease (COPD) is an irreversible airflow limitation commonly caused by inflammatory response of the lungs to exogenous noxious particles or gases (e.g. tobacco smoke). It usually is accompanied by emphysema and chronic bronchitis. COPD causes about 5% of all deaths globally. Its prevalence in the UK is 1–2%. Smoking cessation is the most promising preventive measure. Many sufferers try CAM, particularly herbal medicines.

Clinical bottom line

😊 *Likely to be beneficial*

- Breathing exercises: encouraging evidence from some but not all studies.

😐 *Unknown effectiveness*

- Acupuncture, acupressure: dyspnoea, not enough data available.
- Biofeedback: lung function, not enough data available.
- Chinese herbal mixtures: not enough data available.
- Ginseng (*Panax ginseng*): lung function, not enough data available.
- Guided imagery: may increase oxygen saturation but not enough data available.
- Ivy (*Hedera helix*) leaf extract: dyspnoea, not enough data available.
- Reflexology: not enough data available.
- Relaxation: dyspnoea, not enough data available.

🗙 *Likely to be ineffective or harmful*

- Pomegranate (*Punica granatum*) juice: studies negative.

Conclusions

- Breathing exercises are likely to alleviate symptoms when used with conventional care
- No serious adverse effects known
- The risk–benefit balance for breathing exercises is likely to be positive
- Conventional physiotherapeutic muscle training programmes are effective and drug treatments can alleviate symptoms. Compared to that, CAM seems to have little to offer to COPD sufferers

Further reading

Guo R, Pittler MH, Ernst E. Herbal medicines for the treatment of COPD: a systematic review. *Eur Respir J* 2006; **28**:330–8.

Pneumonia

Profile

Inflammation of the lungs, caused by infections with viruses, fungi, parasites, or (most frequently) bacteria. This causes partial loss of function which can be life threatening. Symptoms include dyspnœa, chest pain, cough (and) fever. Pneumonia is one of the leading causes of death in the elderly. Prevention (immunization, life-style, physiotherapy) is often the key. Treatment should be directed at the cause, e.g. antibiotics for bacterial infection. CAM is often advocated as an adjunctive strategy.

Clinical bottom line

😑 *Unknown effectiveness*

- Chinese herbal mixtures: not enough data for any one preparation.
- Chisan (mixture of 3 herbs): not enough data available.
- Osteopathy: not enough data available.
- Vitamin C: data contradictory and scarce.
- Zinc: data contradictory.

😡 *Unlikely to be beneficial:*

- Vitamin A: not effective in underweight children.
- Vitamin E: not effective in children.

Conclusions

- No CAM treatment has been shown to be effective
- The treatments in question are not associated with serious risks
- The risk–benefit balance fails to be positive
- Very effective conventional treatments are available. CAM has little to offer in addition and should never be used as an alternative

Further reading

Loeb M. Community acquired pneumonia. *Clin Evid* 2006; **15**:2015–24.

Upper respiratory tract infection

Profile

Infections of the upper respiratory tract, i.e. common cold, sore throat (pharyngitis, laryngitis), tonsillitis, sinusitis, or bronchitis can be caused by viruses (most frequent), bacteria, or fungi. Common cold is the most prevalent condition: it is characterized by runny nose, headache, and general malaise. These infections are extremely common (1–2 per person per year) and disappear usually within 1 week regardless of treatment. Numerous CAM treatments are on offer and most patients have tried several of them.

Clinical bottom line

😊 *Beneficial*

- *Andrographis paniculata*: treatment, most trials show a symptomatic improvement.
- Vitamin C: treatment, modest (about 8%) reduction in duration of symptoms.

😊 *Likely to be beneficial*

- Echinacea (*Echinacea* spp): some evidence that preparations based on the aerial parts of *E. purpurea* might be effective for the early treatment of colds in adults but results not fully consistent.
- Exercise (moderate levels): prevention, moderate reduction of risk of infection suggested.

😐 *Unknown effectiveness*

- Chinese herbs: many herbs exist but data unconvincing.
- Garlic (*Allium sativum*): prevention, not enough data available.
- German chamomile (*Matricaria recutita*): treatment, not enough data available.
- Ginseng (*Panax ginseng*): prevention, not enough data available.
- Herbal mixtures: many exist, few have been rigorously tested, no convincing evidence for any specific mixture.
- Homeopathy: treatment, data conflicting.

😠 *Likely to be ineffective or harmful*

- Probiotics: trial data negative.
- Sesame (*Sesasum indicum*) oil: trial data negative.
- Vitamin C: prevention, trials fail to demonstrate efficacy.
- Vitamin E: prevention and treatment, trials fail to demonstrate efficacy.
- Zinc: treatment, trials fails to demonstrate efficacy.

Table 5.23 Systematic up-to-date reviews of treatments that are beneficial for upper respiratory tract infection

Treatment	Source	No. of trials/ patients	Original conclusion
Andrographis paniculata	Planta Medica 2004; **70**:293–96	N=7/n=896	A. paniculata is superior to placebo in alleviating the subjective symptoms of uncomplicated upper respiratory tract infection
Vitamin C	Cochrane Data base Syst Rev 2004; **4**: CD000980	N=30/n=8000	Modest reduction of symptoms when taken for treatment purposes

Conclusions

- High dose vitamin C reduces duration of symptoms marginally, A. paniculata, E. purpurea and exercise may be of benefit
- No serious risks are associated with these treatments
- The risk–benefit balance for vitamin C is positive, for A. paniculata, E. purpurea and exercise it is tentatively positive
- No conventional treatment convincingly works for upper respiratory tract infections unless they are of bacterial origin (antibiotics). The clinical relevance of the effects of CAM is as questionable as that of most conventional approaches for viral upper respiratory tract infections

Further reading

Carr RR, Nahata MC. Complementary and alternative medicine for upper-respiratory-tract infection in children. Am J Health Syst Pharm 2006; **63**:33–9.

Guo R, Canter PH, Ernst E. Herbal medicines for the treatment of rhinosinusitis: a systematic review. Otolaryngol Head Neck Surg 2006; **135**:496–506.

Vitamin C

What is it?

An essential nutrient required for normal body functioning that cannot be synthesized by the human body. The L-enantiomer of ascorbate

How does it work?

As an antioxidant which protects the body against oxidative stress, it is a co-factor for several enzymatic reactions. It acts as an electron donor for enzymes involved in collagen synthesis, which is disrupted in the vitamin C avitaminosis scurvy

How is it used?

75–90mg daily are recommended. Orally, with normal food intake or as dietary supplement

Are there any risks?

Excessive intake (2g daily and more) may cause diarrhoea

Rheumatology

Back pain

Profile

Back pain has many (often unknown) causes. The pain may be constant or intermittent, local or referred into the legs. It is associated with impaired mobility and function. Back pain is amongst the most common conditions afflicting humans. Around 90% of us experience it at some stage in our lives. Conventionally one differentiates between acute (i.e. less than 12 weeks), subacute, and chronic back pain. Other terms are mechanical, idiopathic, non-specific back pain, or lumbago. Occasionally back pain can be the sign of serious disease such as cancer. Back pain is the most frequent reason for people to try CAM, particularly acupuncture, herbal medicines, massage, chiropractic, and osteopathy.

Clinical bottom line

😃 *Likely to be beneficial*
- Acupuncture: even though data are somewhat contradictory, the totality of the evidence suggests that acupuncture reduces chronic back pain.
- Capsaicin: (topical) seems to reduce pain more than placebo.
- Devil's claw (*Harpagophytum procumbens*): seems an effective symptomatic treatment.
- Massage: most trials suggest pain relief.
- Osteopathic treatments: seems to reduce pain.
- Relaxation: short-term pain relief and functional improvement.
- Willow (*Salix alba*): seems to reduce pain.

⚖️ *Trade off between benefits and harms*
- Spinal manipulation: superior to demonstrably harmful treatments in this condition (e.g. bed rest) or to sham manipulation but not more effective than conventional options (e.g. exercise); upper spinal manipulation has been associated with stroke and death.

😐 *Unknown effectiveness*
- Alexander technique: not enough data available.
- Auriculotherapy: not enough data available.
- Biofeedback: not enough data available.
- Comfrey (*Symphytum officinale*): topical, not enough data available.
- Music therapy: not enough data available.
- Water injections: not enough data available.
- Yoga: not enough data available.

Table 5.24 Systematic up-to-date reviews of treatments that are likely to be beneficial for back pain

Treatment	Source	No. of trials/ patients	Original conclusion
Acupuncture	*Ann Intern Med* 2005; **142**:651–663	N=33/NA	Acupuncture effectively relieves chronic low back pain
Devil's claw	*BMC Complement Altern Med* 2004; **4**:13	N=4/n=505	Strong evidence exists for the use of an aqueous *Harpago phytum* extract
Massage	*Spine* 2002; **27**: 1896–1910	N=8/n=891	Massage might be beneficial for patients with subacute and chronic nonspecific LBP

Conclusions

- Acupuncture, capsaicin, devil's claw, massage, osteopathy, relaxation, spinal manipulation, and willow extracts might all be promising treatments for back pain
- Spinal manipulation can be associated with considerable risks, none of the above other treatments are associated with serious risks
- For these interventions, the risk–benefit balance is therefore positive

Further reading

Gagnier JJ, van Tulder M, Berman B, Bombardier C. Herbal medicine for low back pain. *Cochrane Database Syst Rev* 2006; **2**:CD004504.
van Tulder MW, Koes B, Malmivaara A. Outcome of non-invasive treatment modalities on back pain: an evidence-based review. *Eur Spine J* 2006; **15**(1):S64–81.

Chronic fatigue syndrome

Profile

This syndrome is characterized by severe, disabling fatigue, often accompanied by pain, insomnia, impaired cognitive function, or headache. Its aetiology remains elusive and a range of terms have been used for it: e.g. neurasthenia, post-viral fatigue syndrome, myalgic encephalomyelitis (ME), and yuppie flu. As for most long-term conditions which are not curable with conventional medicine, CAM is frequently employed. Popular treatments are acupuncture and massage.

Clinical bottom line

😑 *Unknown effectiveness*

- Evening primrose (*Oenothera biennis*): the few studies available generated contradictory results regarding symptoms ratings.
- Homeopathy: symptom score seems to improve more than with placebo, but trial data scarce.

😣 *Unlikely to be beneficial*

- Siberian ginseng (*Eleutherococcus senticosus*): the trial data show no symptom relief relative to placebo.
- Magnesium: trials testing the effectiveness of magnesium injections generated contradictory findings.
- Relaxation was not superior to cognitive behaviour therapy in a comparative study.

☠ *Likely to be ineffective or harmful*

- Melatonin, the few studies that are available fail to demonstrate effectiveness.

Conclusions

- No compelling evidence exists for any CAM treatment
- No serious risks have been reported
- The risk–benefit balance fails to be positive for any CAM treatment
- The most effective conventional treatments are exercise and cognitive behaviour therapy. No CAM is supported by nearly as good evidence as these approaches

Further reading

Chambers D, Bagnall AM, Hempel S, Forbes C. Interventions for the treatment, management and rehabilitation of patients with chronic fatigue syndrome/myalgic encephalomyelitis: an updated systematic review. *J R Soc Med* 2006; **99**:506–20.

Fibromyalgia

Profile

Fibromyalgia (also muscular rheumatism or fibrositis) is a rheumatic condition characterized by a very wide range of symptoms e.g. tender points over various muscles, on both sides of the body, with diffuse muscle, joint or bone pain, stiffness, fatigue, and insomnia. Women are more often affected than men (9:1) and there may be a genetic predisposition. Most patients try CAM, particularly massage, dietary regimens, herbal and other supplements, relaxation, and acupuncture.

Clinical bottom line

😃 *Likely to be beneficial*

- Mind–body therapies such as meditation, hypnotherapy, relaxation, guided imagery: may improve self-efficacy, quality of life, and pain.

😐 *Unknown effectiveness*

- Acupuncture: data methodologically weak and contradictory.
- Biofeedback: data have methodological limitations.
- Capsaicin: not enough data available.
- Feldenkrais: not enough data available.
- Homeopathy: not enough data available.
- Hydrotherapy, Stangerbad: might improve tender points but not enough data available.
- Magnet therapy: may reduce pain but not enough data available.
- Massage: may improve pain, depression, and quality of life but not enough data available.
- Music therapy: not enough data available.
- Osteopathy: not enough data available.
- Therapeutic touch: not enough data available.

😠 *Likely to be ineffective or harmful*

- Chiropractic: no convincing data for effectiveness and considerable risk of harm.

Table 5.25 Systematic up-to-date review of treatment that is likely to be beneficial for Fibromyalgia

Treatment	Source	No. of trials/ patients	Original conclusion
Mind–body therapies	*J Rheumatol* 2000; **27**:2911–18	N=13/n=802	Mind-body therapies are more effective for some clinical outcomes compared to waiting list/ treatment as usual or placebo. Compared to active treatments, results are largely inconclusive, except for moderate/high intensity exercise, where results favor the latter

Conclusions

- Mind–body therapies may improve pain and quality of life
- These approaches are not associated with serious risks
- Their risk–benefit ratio is therefore positive
- Exercise therapy seems to be more effective than mind–body therapies

Further reading

Sarac AJ, Gur A. Complementary and alternative medical therapies in fibromyalgia. *Curr Pharm Des* 2006; **12**:47–57.

Gur A. Physical therapy modalities in management of fibromyalgia. *Curr Pharm Des* 2006; **12**:29–35.

Neck pain

Profile

Pain in the cervical region is a frequent complaint. It is often associated with referred pain into the shoulders, arms, or head and a loss of mobility. There are many causes for neck pain e.g. degenerative disorders of the soft tissues, osteoarthritis of the cervical spine, and connective tissue diseases. The condition tends to become chronic. Many sufferers try CAM; popular treatments are acupuncture, chiropractic, massage, and osteopathy.

Clinical bottom line

☺ *Beneficial*

- Acupuncture: improves neck pain and disability.

😐 *Unknown effectiveness*

- Massage: trial data demonstrate both positive and negative results for pain control. A Cochrane review concluded that 'the effectiveness of massage for neck pain remains uncertain'.
- Relaxation: compared with usual care, applied relaxation was associated with better pain relief but data is scarce.
- Spa therapy: may improve pain yet not enough data available.

🗶 *Likely to be ineffective or harmful*

- Spinal manipulation/mobilization: as a sole treatment it is not demonstrably effective and associated with serious complications e.g. stroke and death.

Table 5.26 Systematic up-to-date review of treatments that are beneficial for neck pain

Treatment	Source	No. of trials/ patients	Original conclusion
Acupuncture	*Cochrane Database Syst Rev* 2006; **3**:CD004870	N=10/n=661	Moderate evidence that acupuncture relieves pain better than some sham treatments.

Conclusions

- Acupuncture is beneficial for improving pain and disability in the short-term. Long-term effects are less certain
- Administered by a qualified practitioner acupuncture is a relatively safe treatment
- The risk–benefit balance for acupuncture is positive
- The effectiveness of acupuncture relative to conventional treatments (e.g. physiotherapeutic exercise) is uncertain

Further reading

Binder AI. Cervical spondylosis and neck pain. *BMJ* 2007; **334**:527–31.

Acupuncture

What is it?

Treatment from TCM, usually with needle insertion at acupuncture points

How does it work?

In TCM, it is assumed that acupuncture restores the balance of yin and yang. Modern theories are based on neurophysiological concepts such as endorphin release or gate-control therapy

How is it used?

In TCM it is used as a panacea: in 'Western' acupuncture mainly for pain

Are there any risks?

Mild adverse effects occur in about 10% of patients, serious complications (e.g. pneumothorax) are rare

Osteoarthritis

Profile

Osteoarthritis is a degenerative disease of the joints and variously defined by clinical and/or radiological features. It most commonly affects knees, hips, hands, and spinal apophyseal joints. It is characterized by focal areas of damage to the cartilage surfaces of synovial joints and is associated with remodelling of the underlying bone and mild synovitis. Clinical features include pain, bony tenderness, and crepitus. Knee osteoarthritis is about twice as prevalent as hip osteoarthritis in people aged over 60 years. In a general practice setting 1% of people aged over 45 years have a clinical diagnosis of knee osteoarthritis. Risk factors are obesity, abnormalities in joint shape, injury, and previous joint inflammation. Acupuncture, massage, manipulation, and homeopathy are most commonly used.

Clinical bottom line

☺ Beneficial

- Acupuncture: alleviates pain particularly from knee osteoarthritis.
- Phytodolor: a proprietary herbal mixture shown to be safe and effective for alleviating pain and restoring function.

☺ Likely to be beneficial

- Avocado/soybean unsaponifiables: positive but not fully convincing data for symptom control.
- Chondroitin, glucosamine: data suggested effectiveness for pain and function but are contradicted by more recent studies of sulphate and hydrochloride variants; may even prevent joint space narrowing in osteoarthritis.
- Devil's claw (*Harpagophytum procumbens*): moderate evidence suggests pain reduction associated with osteoarthritis of the spine, hip, and knee
- SK1 306X: this mixture of three herbs may be effective for pain relief
- Spa therapy: may alleviate pain and function but data are not entirely convincing.

☺ Unknown effectiveness

- Arnica (*Arnica montana*), herbal tincture: may be effective for improving pain and function in hand osteoarthritis but not enough data available.
- Arthritis Relief Plus: a herbal ointment may improve pain and stiffness yet not enough data available.
- Capsaicin: might be effective in reducing pain but not enough data available.
- Chiropractic: may alleviate back pain secondary to osteoarthritis but not enough data available.
- Comfrey (*Symphytum officinale*): may improve pain and function but not enough data available.
- Duhuo Jisheng Wan: this Chinese herbal mixture may improve pain and stiffness yet not enough data available.
- Ginger (*Zingiber officinalis*): data not convincing for pain relief.

- Gitadyl: some positive evidence yet not enough data available.
- Green lipped muscle (*Perna canaliculus*): little consistent and compelling evidence.
- Herbomineral formulation: some positive evidence yet not enough data available.
- Homeopathy: not enough data for symptom improvement available.
- Hyben vital: some positive evidence yet not enough data available.
- Imagery: may improve quality of life but not enough data available.
- Indian frankincense (*Boswellia serrata*): may reduce pain and increase walking distance yet data scarce with methodological limitations.
- Magnets, static: no compelling evidence for pain relief.
- Massage: may improve pain, stiffness, function, range of motion, but not enough data available.
- Music therapy: not enough data available.
- Reumalex: herbal mixture which may have analgesic effects.
- Rose hip (*Rosa canina*): may reduce pain but more data required.
- Sierrasil: this herbomineral formulation may reduce pain but not enough data available.
- Soy: may alleviate symptoms yet not enough data available.
- Stinging nettle (*Urtica dioica*): may reduce pain in patients with osteoarthritis of the fingers but not enough data available.
- Tai chi: improvement of pain and function, no exacerbation of symptoms but not enough data available.
- Therapeutic touch: not enough data available.
- Willow bark (*Salix* spp): not enough data available.
- Yoga: not enough data available for pain and function.

😕 *Unlikely to be beneficial*
- Eazmov: this Ayurvedic herbal preparation seems ineffective.

🗙 *Likely to be ineffective or harmful*
- Bromelain: likely to be ineffective in moderate-to-severe osteoarthritis.
- Magnets, electromagnetic: ineffective for pain reduction in patients with knee osteoarthritis.
- Tipi: a herbal combination which is likely to be ineffective.
- Vitamin E: seems ineffective for preventing loss of cartilage in knee osteoarthritis.

Table 5.27 Systematic up-to-date reviews of treatments that are beneficial for osteoarthritis

Treatment	Source	No. of trials/ patients	Original conclusion
Acupuncture	*Rheumatology* 2006; **45**:1331–7	N=3/n=329	Sham-controlled RCTs suggest specific effects of acupuncture for pain control in patients with peripheral joint osteoarthritis
Acupuncture	*Acupunct Med* 2006; **24**:S40–48.	N=13/n=2362	Acupuncture is an effective treatment for osteoarthritis of the knee
Phytodolor	*Rheumatology* 2001; **40**:779–93	N=6/n=322	These trials demonstrate significant results for pain reduction, mobility and NSAID consumption with administration of Phytodolor

Conclusions

- Best evidence supports the use of acupuncture and Phytodolor. A number of other interventions are likely to be beneficial for improving pain and function
- Allergic reactions and herb–drug interactions should be considered as possible adverse events with Phytodolor. Serious adverse events in acupuncture are rare
- The risk–benefit balance for acupuncture and Phytodolor is positive for improving pain and function in osteoarthritis. It is likely to be positive for above mentioned other interventions

Further reading

Hunter DJ, Felson DT. Osteoarthritis. *BMJ* 2006; **332**:639–42.

Acupuncture

What is it?
Treatment from TCM, usually with needle insertion at acupuncture points

How does it work?
In TCM, it is assumed that acupuncture restores the balance of yin and yang. Modern theories are based on neurophysiological concepts such as endorphin release or gate-control therapy

How is it used?
In TCM it is used as a panacea: in 'Western' acupuncture mainly for pain

Are there any risks?
Mild adverse effects occur in about 10% of patients, serious complications (e.g. pneumothorax) are rare

Phytodolor

What is it?
Proprietary medicine containing extracts of aspen (*Populus tremula*), ash (*Fraxinus excelsior*), and European goldenrod (*Solidago virgaurea*)

How does it work?
Analgesic, anti-inflammatory

How is it used?
Orally, 3 to 4 times daily, 20–30 drops

Are there any risks?
Allergic reactions, gastrointestinal complaints

Rheumatoid arthritis

Profile

Rheumatoid arthritis (RA) is a chronic disease, mainly characterized by inflammation of the synovium of peripheral joints and other periarticular tissues. It can lead to long-term joint damage, resulting in chronic pain, loss of function, and disability. Other symptoms include fatigue, weakness, morning stiffness, flu-like symptoms, and muscle pain. Commonly, it starts in the joints of the fingers and wrists and usually is symmetrical. Prevalence ranges between 0.5–1.5% of the general population in industrialized countries. Women are more frequently affected. The exact cause is not known but seems multifactorial in people with genetic susceptibility. Patients often try herbal and non-herbal supplements.

Clinical bottom line

☺ Beneficial
- Omega-3 fatty acids: reduces morning stiffness and number of painful/tender joints.
- Phytodolor: a proprietary herbal mixture is safe and effective for alleviating pain and restoring function.

☺ Likely to be beneficial
- Relaxation: seems to alleviate arthritis pain.
- Spa therapy: seems to alleviate pain and improve quality of life.
- Tai chi: improvement of lower extremity range of motion, no exacerbation of symptoms.

☯ Trade off between benefits and harms
- Thunder god vine (*Triptergium wilfordii*): beneficial effects reported but also associated with considerable risks.

☹ Unknown effectiveness
- Garlic: not enough data available.
- Glucosamine: not enough data available for symptom control.
- Green lipped muscle (*Perna canaliculus*): evidence is inconclusive.
- Homeopathy: data conflicting for pain.
- Hypnotherapy: no rigorous trials exist specifically for this condition.
- Magnets: may alleviate pain yet not enough data available.
- Sativex: a cannabis-based oromucosal spray led to improvements in pain, and quality of sleep but not enough data available.
- Spiritual healing: unclear difference to placebo for arthritic pain.
- Suogudan (*Rodgersia aesculifolia*) improvement of joint pain, swelling and morning stiffness but not enough data available.
- Tong luo kai bi: not enough data available for this Chinese herbal remedy.
- *Uncaria tomentosa*: not enough data available.

☹ Unlikely to be beneficial
- Acupuncture: no effects on number of swollen, tender joints, patient's global assessment and disease activity.
- Elk velvet antler: no difference to placebo in terms of effectiveness and adverse events.

- Feverfew (*Tanacetum parthenium*): no relevant effects on clinical or laboratory parameters.
- Indian frankincense *(Boswellia serrata):* no beneficial effects on pain and swelling.
- Probiotic (*Lactobacillus rhamnosus*): no difference in clinical symptom picture to placebo.
- Willow bark (*Salix* spp): no improvement in pain.

☒ Likely to be ineffective or harmful
- Ayurvedic medicines: data fail to show effectiveness.

Table 5.28 Systematic up-to-date reviews of treatments that are beneficial for rheumatoid arthritis

Treatment	Source	No. of trials/ patients	Original conclusion
Omega-3 fatty acids	*Pain* 2007; **129**: 210–23	N=17/n=823	The results of the present meta-analysis, examining omega-3 PUFA supplementation in patients with rheumatoid arthritis or joint pain secondary to inflammatory bowel disease and dysmen orrhoea, suggest that EPA/DHA supplementation reduces patient assessed joint pain intensity, morning stiffness, number of painful and/or tender joints, and NSAID consumption.
Phytodolor	*Int J Adv Rheumatol* 2004; **2**:22–5	N=10/n=1035	The results of this review clearly demon-strated the efficacy in terms of symptom control of this remedy

Conclusions

- Best evidence supports the use of omega-3 fatty acids and phytodolor. Relaxation, spa therapy, tai chi, and thunder god vine are likely to be beneficial for improving pain and function
- Allergic reactions and herb–drug interactions should be considered as possible adverse events with Phytodolor; thunder god vine is associated with considerable risks
- The risk–benefit balance for omega-3 fatty acids and Phytodolor is positive for improving pain and function. For all other interventions the risk–benefit balance is not fully convincing

Further reading

Emery P. Treatment of rheumatoid arthritis. *BMJ* 2006; **332**:152–5.

Fish oil

What is it?
Omega-3 fatty acids from fatty fish such as mackerel, tuna, trout, and salmon

How does it work?
Anti-inflammatory, cholesterol-lowering, inhibition of platelet aggregation, lowers triglycerides

How is it used?
Healthy adults are recommended to eat oily fish at least twice a week. Fish oil supplements: orally, usually in doses of 0.2g eicosapentaenoic acid (EPA) and 0.1g docosahexaenoic acid (DHA) daily

Are there any risks?
High doses may have harmful effects including an increased risk of bleeding

Phytodolor

What is it?
Proprietary medicine containing extracts of aspen (*Populus tremula*), ash (*Fraxinus excelsior*), and European goldenrod (*Solidago virgaurea*)

How does it work?
Analgesic, anti-inflammatory

How is it used?
Orally, 3 to 4 times daily, 20–30 drops

Are there any risks?
Allergic reactions, gastrointestinal complaints

Shoulder pain

Profile

Shoulder pain is common (1-year prevalence about 1%). It originates from the tissues around the shoulder including the glenohumeral, acromioclavicular, sternoclavicular, subacromial, and scapulothoracic joints. Specific conditions include adhesive capsulitis (frozen shoulder), rotator cuff tear, non-calcified tendinosis, calcific tendinitis, subacromial/subdeltoid bursitis, hemiplegic (post-stroke) shoulder pain, and pain referred from the cervical spine. Conventional treatment can be difficult and lengthy which is why CAM is frequently tried.

Clinical bottom line

😃 *Likely to be beneficial*

- Massage: trial data are encouraging in terms of pain relief.

😶 *Trade off between benefits and harms*

- Spinal manipulation: some but not all studies suggest quicker recovery if it is used as an adjunct to conventional care; upper spinal manipulation has been associated with stroke and death.

😞 *Unknown effectiveness*

- Acupuncture: data contradictory.
- Magnet therapy: preliminary data suggested pain relief.
- Qigong: not enough data available.

Conclusions

- Massage and spinal manipulation may be useful
- Massage is relatively safe; upper spinal manipulation has been associated with stroke and death
- The risk–benefit balance for CAM is likely to be positive for massage therapy
- Conventional treatments such as physiotherapy can be effective provided the cause of the pain is carefully evaluated. Compared to conventional care, CAM has little to offer

Further reading

Stevenson K. Evidence-based review of shoulder pain. *Musculoskeletal Care* 2006; **4**:233–9.

Tennis elbow

Profile

Tennis elbow (lateral epicondylitis), is characterized by pain and tenderness over the lateral epicondyle of the humerus and pain on resisted dorsiflex-ion of the wrist, middle finger, or both. Lateral epicondylitis is a common condition, with peak incidence occurring at 40–50 years of age. Tennis elbow is considered to be an overload injury, typically after minor and often unrecognized trauma of the extensor muscles of the forearm. Despite the name tennis elbow, tennis is a direct cause in only a small number of those with lateral epicondylitis. Although lateral elbow pain is generally self-limiting, symptoms can persist for 2 years or longer. The cost is therefore high, both in terms of lost productivity and healthcare use. Acupuncture is frequently used for this condition.

Clinical bottom line

☺ *Likely to be beneficial*
- Acupuncture: there appears to be short-term pain relief.
- Manipulation: some positive evidence for pain outcomes.

😐 *Unknown effectiveness*
- Massage, deep transverse friction: not enough data available.

😣 *Unlikely to be beneficial:*
- Essential fatty acids: no beneficial effects for pain VAS and maximal grip force.

Conclusions

- Data suggest that acupuncture and elbow manipulation are likely to be beneficial for improving pain. This is based on relatively few data and the evidence is not fully compelling
- Adverse events are generally mild and infrequent
- The risk–benefit balance seems positive for acupuncture and manipulation
- Given the limited options in conventional medicine, acupuncture and elbow manipulation seem worth trying in suitable patients

Further reading

Assendelft W, Green S, Buchbinder R, *et al.* Tennis elbow. *Clin Evid* 2004; **11**:1633–44.
Whaley AL, Baker CL. Lateral epicondylitis. *Clin Sports Med* 2004; **23**:677–91.

Urology

Benign prostatic hyperplasia

Profile

An increase in the size of the prostate through benign glandular and stromal hyperplasia commonly in the middle and lateral lobes of the prostate gland. The enlarged prostate increases pressure on neighbouring structures, primarily urethra and bladder, which leads to symptoms of urinary hesitancy, frequent urination, urinary retention, and increased risk of urinary tract infections. Benign prostatic hyperplasia is the most prevalent of all conditions in aging men, with the population prevalence in the 40–79-year age group estimated at 25%.

Clinical bottom line

☺ Beneficial

- African plum (*Prunus africana*): modestly improves symptoms and urinary flow measures.
- Saw palmetto (*Serenoa repens*): improves symptoms and urinary flow measures.

☺ Likely to be beneficial

- Nettle (*Urtica dioica*): may improve symptoms and urinary flow measures.
- PRO160/120 (*Serenoa repens, Urtica dioica*): may improve symptoms.
- Rye grass pollen (*Secale cereale*): may improve symptoms.

☹ Unknown effectiveness

- Pumpkin seed (*Cucurbita pepo*): not enough data available.

Conclusions

- Best evidence suggests that African plum and saw palmetto are beneficial for benign prostatic hyperplasia. Nettle, the combination preparation PRO160/120, and rye grass pollen are likely to be beneficial but the evidence is not fully convincing
- Allergic reactions should be considered. Saw palmetto may increase bleeding time
- The risk–benefit balance for African plum and saw palmetto is positive, for nettle, PRO 160/120 and rye grass pollen likely to be positive
- Compared to the conventional option finasteride, saw palmetto seems similarly effective

Further reading

Kaplan SA. Medical therapy for benign prostatic hyperplasia: new terminology, new concepts, better choices. *Rev Urol* 2006; **8**:14–22.

Patel AK, Chapple CR. Benign prostatic hyperplasia: treatment in primary care. *BMJ* 2006; **333**:535–9.

African plum (*Prunus africana*)

What is it?
African plum is a tree native to the mountainous regions of sub-Saharan Africa and the Islands of Madagascar, Sao Tome, Fernando Po, and Grand Comore

How does it work?
It seems to have anti-inflammatory and antiproliterative effects. The mechanism of action is not known

How is it used?
Orally as capsules

Are there any risks?
Nausea, abdominal pain. May positively interact with 5 alpha-reductase inhibitors, Saw palmetto or stinging nettle extracts. No long-term safety data available

Saw palmetto (*Serenoa repens*)

What is it?
A dwarf palm, parts used for medicinal purposes are the fruits

How does it work?
Inhibition of 5-alpha-reductase, inhibitory effects on the binding of dihydrotestosterone to androgen receptors in the prostate

How is it used?
As extract in tablets or capsules

Are there any risks?
Allergy, may increase bleeding time

Erectile dysfunction

Profile

Erectile dysfunction is defined as the inability to achieve or maintain an erection sufficient for satisfactory sexual performance. Across all ages there is an estimated prevalence of about 10% making it a common condition, which increases in prevalence to over 50% in men between 50–70 years of age. The causes of erectile dysfunction may be physiological or psychological. There is a strong placebo effect and psychological impotence can often be helped by a number of interventions that the patient believes in. It is also linked with organic conditions such as diabetes and cardiovascular disorders, neurological disorders, pelvic surgery, trauma, and as a consequence of pharmacological treatments.

Clinical bottom line

☺ Beneficial
- Yohimbine: superior to placebo.

☺ Likely to be beneficial
- Ginseng (*Panax ginseng*): may improve rigidity, girth, and patient satisfaction.

☺ Unknown effectiveness
- Acupuncture: but too few data available.
- Biofeedback: inconclusive evidence.
- *Butea superba*: may improve sexual function but too few data available.
- Ginkgo (*Ginkgo biloba*): too few data available.
- Hypnotherapy: may improve sexual function but further data required.

Conclusions

- Best evidence suggests that yohimbine is beneficial for erectile dysfunction. Ginseng is likely to be beneficial but the evidence is not fully convincing
- Yohimbine and ginseng are not associated with serious risks but adverse events have been reported, allergic reactions should be considered
- The risk–benefit balance for yohimbine is favourable and likely to be positive for ginseng
- Compared to conventional invasive interventions, there are obvious advantages. There are no comparative studies with other conventional oral medications such as sildenafil

Further reading

Rees J, Patel B. Erectile dysfunction. *BMJ* 2006; **332**:593.

Yohimbe (*Pausinystalia yohimbe*)

What is it?
A tall evergreen tree, which is native to Central Africa. Yohimbine is the main active constituent of yohimbe bark extract

How does it work?
Alpha-2-adrenoceptor blockade. Rise in sympathetic drive by increasing noradrenaline release and firing rate of noradrenergic nuclei in the central nervous system

How is it used?
Indole alkaloids of which 10–15% are yohimbine

Are there any risks?
Nervous excitation, tremor, irritability, sleeplessness, anxiety, hypertension, hypotension, tachycardia, bronchospasm, gastrointestinal complaints, skin flushing, rash, mydriasis

Urinary tract infection

Profile

Urinary tract infections (UTI) can affect any part of the urinary tract: the kidneys, the ureters, the bladder (cystitis), or the urethra. A UTI is defined by the presence of a pure growth of more than 10^5 colony forming units of bacteria per millilitre of urine but lower counts of bacteria may also be clinically important. Symptoms of UTI include a strong urge to urinate that cannot be delayed which is followed by a sharp pain or burning sensation in the urethra when the urine is released. Often very little urine is released and the urine that is released may be tinged with blood. The urge to urinate recurs quickly and soreness may occur in the lower abdomen, back, or sides. Cranberry juice or tablets are popular herbal remedies for UTI.

Clinical bottom line

☺ *Likely to be beneficial*
- Cranberry (*Vaccinium macrocarpon*): prevention of UTI in women.

☻ *Unknown effectiveness*
- Acupuncture: encouraging results in women but not enough data available.
- Angocin Anti-Infekt: a herbal drug containing nasturtium and horseradish root, not enough data available.
- Cranberry (*Vaccinium macrocarpon*): treatment of UTI, not enough data available.
- Zishen Tongli Jiaonang: Chinese herbal remedy, not enough data available.

✗ *Likely to be ineffective or harmfu*
- Cranberry (*Vaccinium macrocarpon*): ineffective in preventing UTI in patients with neurogenic bladder secondary to spinal cord injury.

Table 5.29 Systematic up-to-date review of treatment that is likely to be beneficial for urinary tract infection

Treatment	Source	No. of trials/ patients	Original conclusion
Cranberry	*Cochrane Database Syst Rev 2004;* **2**: CD001321	N=7/n=604	There is some evidence from two good quality RCTs that cranberry juice may decrease the number of symptomatic UTIs over a 12 month period in women

Conclusions

- There is reasonably good evidence that cranberry juice may be useful in the prevention of UTIs in women but its effects in other populations (e.g. the elderly, children) are unclear
- Cranberry is relatively safe if consumed in recommended doses, diabetics should consider high sugar content of the juice
- The risk–benefit balance for cranberry in preventing UTI in women seems positive
- CAM should not be used instead of antibiotics in manifest infections

Further reading

Franco AV. Recurrent urinary tract infections. *Best Pract Res Clin Obstet Gynaecol 2005*; **19**:861–73.

Miscellaneous conditions

Insomnia

Profile

Sleep problems are common and can relate to poor quality of sleep, frequent awakening, difficulty in falling asleep, or early awakening. Often fear, anxiety, stress, or an unhealthy lifestyle are at the root of primary insomnia. Secondary insomnia is caused by specific medical condition or environmental factors. If these problems occur 3 nights per week for 1 month or longer, we speak of chronic insomnia. Many insomniacs try CAM, particularly relaxation and herbal medicine.

Clinical bottom line

☺ Beneficial

- Melatonin: several trials demonstrate that melatonin improves initial sleep quality, particularly in the elderly.
- Relaxation: results uniformly show that relaxation reduces sleep problems.

☺ Likely to be beneficial

- Autogenic training: trial data positive but scarce.
- Hypnotherapy: trials often methodologically weak but suggest effectiveness.
- Valerian (*Valeriana officinalis*): even though somewhat contradictory, most studies suggest effectiveness.

☺ Trade off between benefits and harms

- Kava (*Piper methysticum*): this anxiolytic herbal medicine has been demonstrated to be effective but is suspected to cause liver damage.

☹ Unknown effectiveness

- Acupuncture: studies methodologically limited and contradictory.
- Aromatherapy: not enough data available.
- Biofeedback: studies contradictory.
- Hops (*Humulus lupulus*): beneficial effects of hops/valerian combination products but role of hops is unclear.
- Massage: not enough data available.
- Music: not enough data available.
- TCM, insomnia in patients with hypertension: not enough data available.
- Yoga, sleep quality: not enough data available.

Table 5.30 Systematic up-to-date review of treatment that is beneficial for insomnia

Treatment	Source	No. of trials/ patients	Original conclusion
Melatonin	*Z Gerontol Geriatr* 2001; **34**:491-497	N=6/95	There is sufficient evidence that low doses of melatonin improve initial sleep quality in selected elderly subjects

Conclusions

- Relaxation, melatonin and kava are effective treatments; autogenic training, hypnotherapy and valerian may be effective
- Relaxation, autogenic training and hypnotherapy are not associated with serious risks. The short-term safety profiles of melatonin and valerian are favourable; kava has been associated with liver damage
- The risk–benefit balance for relaxation and melatonin is positive. For other CAM treatments it may turn out to be positive
- Relaxation is an ideal adjunct to conventional therapy. Whether any CAM intervention is better than conventional treatment is not known

Further reading

Pearson NJ, Johnson LL, Nahin RL. Insomnia, trouble sleeping, and complementary and alternative medicine: Analysis of the 2002 national health interview survey data. *Arch Intern Med* 2006; **166**:1775–82.

Melatonin

What is it?

Melatonin is a neurohormone synthesized from tryptophan. Release is stimulated by darkness and suppressed by light. It is involved in the regulation of bodily rhythms such as temperature and sleep

How does it work?

Synchronising hormone secretion, sedative, antioxidative, immune stimulating, antiproliferative, anti-inflammatory, hypotensive

How is it used?

- Insomnia: 1–2 hours before bedtime
- Jet lag: at 22–2400 hrs local time on arrival for 4 days

Are there any risks?

Abdominal cramps, fatigue, dizziness. May potentiate the effects of benzodiazepines and antihypertensive drugs. May reduce the effects of warfarin and antihyperglycaemic drugs

Relaxation therapy

What is it?
Techniques for eliciting the 'relaxation response' of the autonomic nervous system

How does it work?
Progressive muscle relaxation elicits the relaxation response, resulting in the normalizing of blood supply to the muscles, decreases in oxygen consumption, heart rate, respiration, and skeletal muscle activity and increases in skin resistance and alpha brain waves. Other relaxation techniques involve passive muscle relaxation, refocusing, or breathing

How is it used?
Several months of daily practise is needed in order to be able to evoke the relaxation response

Are there any risks?
None known

Smoking cessation

Profile

Smoking is an addiction and a risk factor for several serious conditions, e.g. arteriosclerosis and cancer. Therefore, it would be hugely important to develop effective cessation programmes. There are numerous claims for CAM being beneficial in this context, and many smokers are persuaded to try CAM, e.g. acupuncture, various herbal and non-herbal supplements, or hypnotherapy.

Clinical bottom line

☺ *Unknown effectiveness*

- Acupressure: not enough data available.
- Massage: withdrawal symptoms may be lessened by massage but trial data scarce.
- Relaxation: may reduce stress during nicotine withdrawal yet not enough data available.

☒ *Likely to be ineffective or harmful*

- Acupuncture: the majority of rigorous studies fail to show an effect on cessation rates over and above a placebo response.
- Hypnotherapy: no convincing evidence compared to other psychological interventions.
- St John's wort: data fail to show that this is an effective aid for smoking cessation.

Conclusions

- No CAM therapy has been shown to be effective
- No serious risks have been reported for the above treatments
- The risk–benefit balance is not positive for any CAM
- Compared to approaches such as nicotine plasters or cognitive behavioural therapy CAM has little to offer

Further reading

Dean AJ. Natural and complementary therapies for substance use disorders. *Curr Opin Psychiatry* 2005; **18**:271–6.

Chapter 6

Vulnerable populations

CAM for children

Prevalence

The prevalence of CAM usage by children is generally similar to that of adults. Asthma, autism, cancer, and eczema are amongst the paediatric conditions most frequently treated with CAM. Herbal medicine, homeopathy, and dietary supplements are the CAM modalities most often used to treat children; massage is commonly used in newborn infants. There is no large, nationally representative survey available for the UK. The American Academy of Pediatrics estimates that 20–40% of healthy children and more than 50% of children with chronic, recurrent, and incurable conditions use CAM. Surveys from Canada and Turkey report CAM use among 49% of paediatric oncology patients and a US survey found that 74% of children with autism used CAM. Survey data also suggest that, if the parents use CAM, their children are likely to also receive it.

An important motivation for parents when choosing CAM is the incorrect notion that CAM is risk-free. Frequently parents do not volunteer information about their child using CAM to their doctor. The above surveys found non-disclosure of CAM use in children to be between 50–66%. It has been noted that CAM use is rarely entered into a child's medical records. Direct questioning is therefore necessary to determine use.

Limited evidence

Paediatrics often relies on extrapolation rather than direct evidence on the effectiveness of medical treatments. If a therapy works in adults, it is usually assumed that it is also effective for children. This applies to conventional healthcare as much as it does for CAM. There are few studies which were actually conducted in a paediatric population. This may be understandable; the ethics of conducting clinical trials with children are generally more complex, but it is nonetheless regrettable and increases the already considerable level of uncertainty we encounter in CAM.

However, some CAM modalities are supported by reasonably good data:
- Probiotics for preventing diarrhoea of diverse causes.
- Probiotics for reducing the symptoms of eczema in children.
- Acupuncture and acupressure for reducing post-operative nausea and vomiting in children.
- Hypnotherapy for improving procedure-related pain, anxiety, as well as nausea and vomiting in paediatric oncology patients.

Safety

Safety is obviously an important issue. Children are not small adults but differ from them, for example, in how their bodies absorb, use, and eliminate medications and other substances. Their immune and central nervous systems are not fully developed, which can make them (especially infants and young children) respond to treatments differently than adults. The common perception that CAM is, almost by definition, harmless and therefore safe for children is certainly not true.

Oral treatments

With any form of CAM taken by mouth, we must consider that a child's metabolism might not be as mature as that of an adult, and certainly, due to the relatively lower body weight, the dose needs careful consideration. In principle, the same rules as those of conventional paediatric pharmacologic medical therapy apply.

Physical treatments

Depending on a child's age, their physical structure and strength has to be taken account of. This has implications for a range of CAM modalities, e.g.:

- Joint manipulations should not be performed before bone structures are strong enough to resist the forces involved.
- Massage therapists have to adjust their technique accordingly.
- Acupuncturists have to consider the different anatomical situation in children.

Mind–body therapies

These treatments usually require a fully developed central nervous system, concentration, and self-control. In very young children they are therefore contraindicated.

Immunization

Immunization is an obvious area of concern. Numerous studies have shown that some CAM practitioners advise parents against immunizing their children. Such advice not only jeopardizes the health of that particular child, it also endangers herd immunity and could, if widespread, bring back epidemics long thought to be a thing of the past. Healthcare professionals should be aware of the attitude of some CAM providers towards immunization and advise the child's parents accordingly.

CAM for the elderly

Prevalence

Although research indicates that chronic health conditions and disability, to which the elderly are naturally more susceptible, are predictors of CAM use, older people's CAM use has been little studied. The 2002 US National Health Interview Survey including the Alternative Health Supplement suggests that use is high in elderly patients with certain conditions; it reports that among adults aged 65 or over almost 70% of those with hypertension and over 80% of those with anxiety or depression used CAM for any indication. Representative data for CAM use among the general elderly population are not available but it is likely to be high.

Evidence and safety

Little of the clinical evidence on CAM has been derived from studying elderly patients. Usually we extrapolate trial data from one age group to another: if it works in the middle-aged or younger individuals we assume that it is also effective in the elderly. However, we must consider reduced metabolic rate and impaired organ function which are more frequent in the elderly. This may require careful adjustment of doses of herbal medicines, for instance. A further important consideration may be herb–drug interactions. Elderly patients are more likely to take prescription drugs than younger ones. This increases the risk of herb–drug interactions. A complete medical history (not just of elderly patients) should include questions about CAM use—we know from numerous surveys that many patients fail to volunteer such information. Osteoporosis is particularly common in the elderly, especially in women. This has important implications for a range of physical CAM approaches. Vigorous spinal manipulation, for instance, is contraindicated in patients with severe osteoporosis. Even vigorous massage can lead to bone fractures in such cases.

CAM options for common ailments in the elderly

CAM options which are supported by good evidence exist for some of the conditions that are typical for elderly patients.

Herbal and non-herbal medicines

- *Ginkgo biloba* can improve cognition and function and delays the clinical course of dementias.
- Guar gum (*Cyamopsis tetragonolobus*) and psyllium (*Plantago ovata*) can reduce total and LDL cholesterol levels in diabetic patients.
- Horse chestnut (*Aesculus hippocastanum*) seed extract is an efficacious and safe short-term treatment for chronic venous insufficiency.
- Melatonin improves initial sleep quality, particularly in the elderly.
- Omega-3 fatty acids reduce pain intensity, morning stiffness, and number of painful/tender joints in rheumatoid arthritis.
- Saw palmetto (*Serenoa repens*) and African plum (*Prunus africana*) can improve the symptoms of benign prostatic hyperplasia.
- St John's wort (*Hypericum perforatum*) is effective in mild-to-moderate depression.

- The proprietary herbal mixture Phytodolor is safe and effective in alleviating pain and restoring function in osteoarthritis and rheumatoid arthritis.
- Yohimbine is effective for erectile dysfunction.

Complementary therapies
- Acupuncture alleviates pain particularly from knee osteoarthritis.
- Biofeedback can lower systolic and diastolic blood pressure.
- There is an encouraging body of evidence that tai chi is safe and effective in promoting balance control and flexibility, and reduces the fear of falling in older people.

Conclusion

In conclusion, many forms of CAM have considerable potential for elderly patients. CAM-providers should, however, have experience in treating the elderly and carefully consider the special needs and particular risks.

CAM during pregnancy and lactation

As most pharmacological treatments are not an option during pregnancy and lactation, many women perceive CAM as an attractive alternative. CAM is wrongly considered to be 'natural' and therefore risk-free. There is, however, still very little reliable information on the safety of CAM available, especially when used during pregnancy. This is particularly relevant for herbal medicines. Some herbal medicines have known constituents or pharmacological activities which make them documented or at least reputed abortifacients. In the present handbook, the precautionary principle has been applied and pregnancy and lactation are listed as contraindications for all medicines unless evidence of safety has been reliably established.

It is nevertheless likely that the demand for CAM to treat general and pregnancy-related complaints will continue and that many women will use CAM without informing their health care professional. Conclusive prevalence data of CAM use during pregnancy in the UK are not available but surveys from other countries suggest that between 40% (e. g. United Arab Emirates) and 60% (e.g. Australia, Canada) of women use some form of CAM during pregnancy. Between 7% (US) and 36% (Norway) are reported to use herbal remedies during pregnancy.

Evidence and safety of CAM treatments popular during pregnancy

Popular CAM treatments during pregnancy include ginger and acupuncture/acupressure to treat nausea and vomiting as well as raspberry leaf or homeopathic preparations for the induction of labour.

Herbal medicines

The use of ginger (*Zingiber officinale*) for pregnancy-related nausea and vomiting is supported by good evidence and there is encouraging safety data which, however, needs to be confirmed in further studies.

Raspberry (*Rubus idaeus*) leaf is a popular herbal remedy but the preliminary evidence of its ability to accelerate the second stage of labour needs to be confirmed in further studies. No systematic safety data exist and concentrated raspberry leaf preparations are likely to be unsafe because they may initiate labour.

Homeopathy

Caulophyllum is a commonly used homeopathic remedy to induce labour. The evidence for it and other homeopathic preparations for third trimester ripening or labour induction is, however, insufficient to recommend them as a method of induction. Safety of homeopathy during pregnancy and lactation has not been assessed systematically but it is unlikely that highly diluted homeopathic preparations would cause adverse effects in mothers or fetuses.

Acupuncture and acupressure

The stimulation of acupoints through acupuncture, acupressure, or electrical devices is used to control pain, induce labour, and to reduce pregnancy-related nausea and vomiting. Although there is encouraging evidence for acupuncture as an adjunct to conventional pain control, there is not enough data available to make any recommendations. Insufficient evidence is available for induction of labour. Finger or wristband acupressure as well as electrical acupoint stimulation are effective in reducing nausea and vomiting while the data for acupuncture remains contradictory. If administered by a responsible acupuncturist, acupoint stimulation is relatively safe and is useful for treating pregnancy-related nausea and vomiting.

Other CAM treatments

Hypnosis, immersion in water, intracutaneous sterile water injections, and massage seem to be useful in reducing pain during labour and are not associated with serious safety concerns.

Conclusion

CAM treatments seem attractive options during pregnancy and lactation and there is evidence to support the use of some of them. Safety is however of paramount importance and pregnant and breastfeeding women should always be advised of the risks associated with CAM use.

Chapter 7

Frequently asked questions

What is the difference between 'complementary' and 'alternative' medicine?

Although the terms are used interchangeably by some, they do have distinct meanings. Alternative medicine was a term popular in the 1980s and defined modalities used instead of conventional medicine. Complementary medicine refers to treatments that are used alongside conventional medicine.

Where can I find reliable advice on CAM?

Be very wary of information gleaned from the internet. There is a vast amount of information available but only a small fraction comes from reliable and trustworthy sources. The Information resources chapter (📖 see p.32–35) provides details of websites, databases, journals, and organizations that provide reliable information about CAM. In addition, a very good way of finding peer reviewed, good quality information is to use the online website evaluation service Intute *www.intute.ac.uk*

How can I find a good therapist?

It is important to find a well qualified therapist. Details on practitioner qualifications can be found in the The regulation of CAM chapter (📖 p.16–19). For NHS health professionals the NHS health directory *http://www.nhsdirectory.org* contains a searchable database of CAM practitioners. For patients and non-NHS health professionals it is best to approach the respective CAM organizations. Most therapies have their own organizations with lists of qualified practitioners. The NHS CAM specialist library provides a list of professional organizations by therapy: *www.library.nhs.uk/cam*

My chiropractor is a doctor; does that mean she has studied medicine?

No. In the UK anyone can legally call themselves a doctor so long as they do not claim to falsely have a PhD or be registered with the General Medical Council. Some chiropractors hold a post graduate diploma in Doctor of Chiropractic (DC) but can not claim to be medical doctors. Further information on this can be found on the General Chiropractic Council's website *www.gcc-uk.org*

How do I know which brand of herbal medicine to buy?

Ask your doctor or pharmacist—they should be able to help you. Generally, it is best to buy only products from well known, reputable companies.

Are there any adverse effects to CAM?

Yes, contrary to popular belief, CAM is not risk-free and can be associated with adverse effects. Some therapies, for example many of the mind–body therapies, are relatively safe when administered by an adequately qualified and responsible therapist. Others are, however, associated with adverse effects and can interact with other medication. Physical injuries may be observed following acupuncture leading in rare cases to pneumothorax or spinal injury. Complications after acupuncture, resulting from infection include hepatitis. Allergic reactions have been reported for a range of herbal and non-herbal medicines. Toxicity has been associated with various herbal preparations involving the liver, kidneys, and the heart. Some herbs may have properties that can cause cancer. You should always inform yourself about any potential risks associated with CAM use.

My GP has no patience with CAM therefore I don't tell him I use it. Is that OK?

No, you should always tell your GP if you use CAM because it might interact with any other medication you are taking. In general, your GP needs to know about any treatment you are using so they can treat you optimally.

Can I use CAM alongside my regular medicine?

If you are using herbal or non-herbal supplements it is best to avoid taking them alongside your regular medicine unless they have been recommended by your GP. Interactions between the supplement and your medicine may have unwanted effects. It is important that you inform your doctor that you are taking supplements.

I am pregnant, can I use CAM?

CAM is not entirely risk-free and particularly during pregnancy and lactation the precautionary principle should be applied. Some herbal and non-herbal supplements can have abortifacient properties; others should not be used during pregnancy and lactation because reliable safety data are missing. Orally taken medicines are therefore contraindicated in pregnancy unless compelling evidence of safety is available. Other forms of CAM, for example mind–body therapies such as yoga, qigong, and tai chi can normally be safely practised during pregnancy if extreme postures are avoided and they are taught by a responsible therapist (📖 see also Vulnerable populations, p.410–411).

Can my child use CAM?

Children can in principle use CAM but safety is an important issue. CAM should not be considered as naturally risk-free and therefore safe for children. For any orally taken CAM, it needs to be taken into account that a child's metabolism is not as mature as that of an adult and doses need adjusting. The physical structure and strength of a child has implications for manipulative therapies. Mind–body therapies require a fully developed central nervous system and self-control and might not be suitable for young children. There are few data on the effectiveness of CAM in children available and most are extrapolated from adult populations (📖 see also Vulnerable populations, p.406–407)

If a treatment has been used for hundreds of years, do we really need trials to prove its effectiveness and safety?

Yes. History has shown that some treatments employed for a long time turned out to be useless or harmful when tested in clinical trials. Decisions on whether to use CAM treatments should be based on the findings of rigorous research. Only then may a CAM treatment be deemed effective and safe.

If I feel better after using CAM, why do I need 'evidence'?

Many factors can contribute to make you feel better when using CAM, which does not necessarily has to be the treatment itself. It could, for instance, be the additional attention you receive. It is important to know whether the actual treatment caused the improvement. For this to know evidence from rigorous clinical trials is required.

How can you say that a particular treatment is probably just a placebo? I've improved!

Placebo or non-specific effects (that is effects not directly related to the treatment) come in many forms and no-one is immune to those non-specific effects. If a treatment, for instance homeopathy, consistently shows improvements in patients suffering from a particular condition but fails to show those improvements in trials that are more rigorous (i.e. exclude bias and error to a greater extent) it is likely that the treatment is a placebo. Placebo is nothing negative. In fact, it can have quite powerful and beneficial effects. However, placebo or non-specific effects come with every treatment irrespective of what the treatment actually entails—and usually it is free!

Isn't the reason why there are so many negative trials because CAM needs to be researched differently?

The need for rigorous testing is often denied by CAM advocates arguing that the randomized clinical trial cannot capture the subtle effects of CAM. The whole reason for testing a treatment in a trial is to find out whether it is effective—in other words, whether it has specific properties that are causing an improvement in a patient. Because bias and error produce misleading results in clinical trials and may lead to false decisions in clinical practice, certain features are included in trials that eliminate such biases and errors (e.g. randomization, control group etc.). If a treatment, whether it be CAM or conventional, has effects that are too subtle to show up in results of rigorous trials then this treatment is unlikely to be beneficial for the patient.

Isn't one reason why CAM has little support is that Big Pharma is suppressing it?

Today CAM has substantial public support; that was different 10 years ago. There is no evidence that the pharmaceutical industry is suppressing CAM. In fact, CAM receives considerable support from many companies.

Index

The term 'complementary medicines' has been abbreviated to CMs.